I AM NOT FAT

how to cope with obesity and live freely

Abe Solyman

Copyright © 2021 Abdelrahman Soliman (Abe Solyman)

All rights reserved

I have tried to recreate events, locales and conversations from my memories of them. In order to maintain their anonymity in some instances I have changed the names of individuals and places, I may have changed some identifying characteristics and details such as physical properties, occupations and places of residence.

No part of this book may be reproduced, or stored in a retrieval system, or transmitted in any form or by any means, electronic, mechanical, photocopying, recording, or otherwise, without express written permission of the publisher.

ISBN-13: 978-0-578-83480-1
ISBN-10: 0-578-83480-1

Printed in the United States of America

To my friends and family, and a special dedication to my four monkeys; my niece, Nour, and my nephews, Islam, Zein and Malek

CONTENTS

Title Page
Copyright
Dedication
A Message Dear to My heart — 1
Part One — 7
The Day I Have Been Waiting For — 8
After the Tryouts — 15
Years from Hell — 26
A New School. A New Beginning, Or Not — 38
Third Time's a Charm — 52
Parkour: Pursuing A Buried Passion — 58
The Accident — 69
Part Two — 76
The Turning Point — 77
Life Changing Decision — 87
The Worst Thing in Life Can Become The Best Thing in Life — 92

Food Addiction — 97
Why Did The Diet Work? — 104
Mental Games — 111
The Victimhood Syndrome — 115

EgyCon – My Fairytale	118
A Dream Came to Life: My First Talk	128
How I Became a Young Entrepreneur?	137
The Fall of SWAT	147
I am not clingy…I swear	156
Falling Down the Slippery Slope	169
Rise of The Phoenix	173
Karma, is that you?	179
Part Three	182
Don't Judge People By Their Social Media Cover.	183
Unfair and Unrealistic Comparisons	186
Unachievable Standards	189
Bad Days Happen to Good People	193
It's Not the End of The Journey, But the Beginning of A New One.	200
APPENDIX	205
What SWAT Taught Me	206
Entrepreneurial Lessons	209
ACKNOWLEDGMENTS	211

A MESSAGE DEAR TO MY HEART

We often cross paths with people who make a difference and leave a mark in our lives. And when we go our separate ways, we wonder how our lives would have turned out had we not met them. Abdel Rahman Soliman belongs to these people. I am in a better place today because of him. We met at the end of the summer of 2016. He became a force of change in my life. I was 16 and I had a tough childhood because of my obesity. Abdel Rahman's journey of transformation both inspired and motivated me. To date, I consider it the most powerful influence that changed my life.

    I related to Abdel Rahman's childhood. It strikingly resembled mine. Growing up obese, neither of us played any sports nor had a healthy social life. We were bullied by just about everyone we met. Abdel Rahman, however, changed his circumstances and made me believe I could change mine as well, which I did.

    By the time I joined SWAT[1], I had tried and failed to lose weight many times. At the beginning of every summer, I dieted, on my own or with dietitians. I joined gyms, hired personal trainers, but nothing worked. SWAT attracted me because it was an independent entity, not affiliated with any gym, no equipment needed. Calisthenics workout was still a novelty in Egypt; flips, muscle up, back lever, front lever. Abdel Raham mastered the bar. He bar-danced swiftly. The thought that one day I could lose weight and bar-dance like him fascinated me. He inspired me to follow his suit.

The spirit of SWAT's team, both trainers and trainees, highly contributed to my weight loss success. We all supported and encouraged each other. We were almost the same age and this created a feeling of bondage, a camaraderie between the team members. I joined many gyms before and they lacked this spirit. Becoming a member of an extended team and exercising together made all the difference.

My commitment to the team and desire to succeed paid off. For the first time in my life I witnessed changes happening to me; noticeable weekly improvements. Not only my weight dropped, which of course became a driving force, but I also witnessed a gradual overall self-improvement, that replaced my old self with a new one, on the physical, emotional and mental levels. My training performance improved, as well as my health and self confidence. This prompted me to continue.

Unlike many trainers who neither motivated me nor believed I could lose weight, often discouraged me to even try, Abdel Rahman helped me throughout my weight loss journey. He encouraged and supported me, always had my back. He pushed me to succeed and helped me fight my demons and insecurities. He understood what I went through, for he traveled the exact journey and made an enormous transformation in his life. His encouragement and support came from his deep belief in me that I can do it.

With SWAT, I dropped from 120kg to 78kg in eight and a half months, a total of 40kgs. Regretfully, with my busy school schedule studying for my IGCSE diploma, I cut down on training. With no time to prepare the healthy food I needed to sustain my weight loss, I gradually fell back to my old routine. It took me two years to gain back some of the weight I had lost.

Abdel Rahman's story not only resonated with me, but also with every child suffering from obesity. Perhaps children do not understand how obesity affects their lives until they are older and they compare their childhood with their peers. Only then they realize how different their childhoods were and how their weight had restricted them from engaging in activities like other children their age. Obese children are deprived of the childhood fun that non-obese children enjoy and take for granted.

I could not go on certain rides in amusement parks. I did

not have play dates. Girls wouldn't look at me. I could not even play hide and seek, for crying out loud! Even sitting on the school bench was uncomfortable. I missed a lot in my life because of my weight. Not to mention how everyone bullied me; children my age, older children, younger children, the teachers, and everyone in between. Their jokes and comments frustrated and angered me. Even if they didn't mean them in a demeaning way to upset me, their jokes hurt and humiliated me.

Abdel Rahman understood all that. He saved me from myself, from the harm I would have caused myself because of my obesity; emotionally or physically. He saved me from the severe depression I had fallen in, and the suicide thoughts that accompanied it. I am also in better health because of him.

I consider Abdel Rahman the most influential person in my life. I changed because of him, and as a result my life improved. He changed my mindset. He instilled in me a new one I didn't know existed. Because of him, I learned how to become a fighter, not just to lose weight, but also to pursue my life goals. I learned that if I set a goal, I will reach it if I work hard towards it. He taught me dedication, commitment, and sacrifice. I learned to sacrifice many things to reach my goal.

Abdel Rahman, you changed my life, man, my way of thinking and more. Keep going, keep changing lives, the world needs people like you.

Thanks for everything you did for me.

Mohamed Khafagy
December 2, 2020

My name is Abdel Rahman Soliman.
My friends call me, Abe Solyman,
and this is my story

PART ONE
Welcome to My World

THE DAY I HAVE BEEN WAITING FOR

I dodged the traffic towards the entrance of the club, moving even a step faster than Karim, lingering behind and talking on his mobile phone, probably planning an outing with his friends later tonight. An outing I was not invited to. The hot asphalt shimmered and radiated heat. It felt soft, almost melting under my feet, like walking on the moon. With all the positive vibes and energy that filled me, I might as well have been walking on the moon, floating in space, reaching out to grab some stars and claim them mine.

The dense air loaded with fumes and car exhausts smelled of tar and gasoline. It hit me in the face, already irritated from the sweat and heat. The cars burnt to the touch. With the exercise bag on my shoulder, I swiftly cut between the cars with lightness that even surprised me. Cars honked at me. Drivers yelled and made fun of me. I did not care.

I reached the other side and waited by the gate. I wiped my forehead with the back of my hand and urged Karim to hurry up. The traffic light turned green for pedestrians. He maneuvered his way through traffic and caught up with me. I have made this journey a thousand times from my home to the club before, but today it was different.

Engaged in a heated conversation, hotter than the air temperature, the guards by the entrance greeted us nonchalantly, raising their arms halfway waving at us, without looking in our direction. We knew they saw and recognized us; faces and names. We make this trip at least once a day. They never stopped us and we never had to show our club membership cards, mine tucked safely in my wallet.

We walked towards the basketball court. My strides longer and faster, as if propelled by my racing heartbeats. The club was crowded with its members. Despite the heat, the club members carried on with their activities, not to miss a moment of action if they could afford to. After all, most people were already on the beaches, elsewhere, enjoying their summer vacations. Children screeched and chased each other. A lazy cat with emerald green eyes watched them from under the shade of a tree, lazily stretching its body, on alert to run away if they approached.

My heart throbbed and my excitement soared with every step toward our destination. We had arrived a few minutes before our meeting. Karim lingered behind as usual, greeting this and chatting with that. I tried to contain myself, but I could not wait for him any longer. I continued my walk to the basketball court. The court already looked like a beehive. Players buzzing around in all directions, loud, sweaty, out of breath. Our peers at the junior basketball academy sat outside the court watching them. Everybody waited anxiously. It was our big day. My big day. The day I have been waiting and working hard for, for three years.

Players ran from one side of the court to the other. Some dribbling balls, others shooting hoops. Some balls hit the rim and bounced back. Tall guys dunked it with ease and made sure everybody watched. Everyone was shouting. A ball flew from somewhere and hit a player in the face, real hard. He staggered, lost his balance and fell to the ground. An older player from the professional team, who assisted the coach during the summer time, refereed the game. The young referee blew his whistle, raised his hand and yelled at the boy who threw the ball. For everyone it was another training day. For me, a start of a new phase in my life, like graduation day. I was about to graduate from the junior basketball academy and join the professional team of Dokki Shooting Club. At fourteen, that made me feel like an adult.

Our coach, Captain Hanafy, approached. We made eye contact and he waved at me. I waved back. He gave me a subtle smile and a nod of reassurance. I smiled back. His sight filled me with relief and hope. He was more than a coach to me, a mentor, an older brother, maybe even closer than my own. He saw my potential when no one else did. He put me under his wing. After the training sessions ended, he allowed me to stay longer and train alone to improve my skills. We had worked hard together for this moment. I had worked really hard for this moment. With his guidance and assistance, I made the cut at every try-out at the junior academy. Prior to basketball I had lost hope I would ever play a sport, let alone enjoy one. When I discovered basketball, I clung to it. I lived at a walking distance from the club, and I haven't missed a day of training for the past three years. And during this time I had improved a lot.

Few steps behind Hanafy, Captain Mourad walked towards us. Taller than most of the crowd, the former basketball player, and current technical director of the professional team was visible to everyone. In the heat of August, he still wore his black coat. He wore it in winters and summers over his training suit pants. With his eyes covered with dark shades, he walked with an aura around him, his two assistants by his side, each carrying a clipboard with a notepad. Whistles dangling around their necks, their trade marks.

Captain Hanafy worked under Mourad and coached the junior academy. He scouted for the new crop of players every year. Hanafy blew his whistle, louder and longer than usual. It pierced our ears and caught everyone's attention. Silence befell on the noisy court.

Of all the sports my mother forced me to play as a child, I liked basketball. Even though I could not run fast when I first joined the junior academy, surprisingly I had good shooting skills. It was the first sport I actually knew how to play and achieved good results at it. To be honest, when I first joined I was not passionate about the game and did not take it seriously the first three years. But during these years, the club hired Captain Hanafy who saw some potential in me and gave me the opportunity to improve. I loved the sport because of him.

Mourad towered over the children like a general in the army. He came today with one mission, to select the new cadets. I never had the chance to talk to him in person before. He coached the professional team I was about to join. Tens of junior players surrounded him, Karim already lost in the crowd. I saw him last standing with some of the cool boys in the academy where he perfectly fit.

The technical director started sorting out the crop. He nodded in the direction of this and that, exchanged smiles with this and that, padded the shoulders of this and that. His assistants wrote down or crossed off names in their writing pads. The ones selected stood on their right side, Karim among them.

Captain Hanafy nodded at me. Time to meet the general.

I stood up straight like a proud soldier would, and approached him cautiously, inhaling deeply to calm down my heart, ready to jump out of my chest. Joining the professional team would be my dream come true. Other than my unconditional passion for basketball, I was thrilled to belong to a team, be part of an extended family, part of something. Joining the team meant I will have friends. I will bond with them. I was already dreaming of all the fun things we were going to do together; join the training camps, travel and play games. I will finally have the chance to live like the rest of the boys I always admired, and envied. For the first time in my life, I felt my dreams will finally come true. My hopes were high. I had no doubt I would make it to the cut. I had given basketball training 110 percent of my time, money and effort, to improve my skills, and it had certainly paid off so far.

As I walked closer I waited for the smile Mourad had showered the other children with, a nod, or a recognition of any sort, but all I received was a stern expression. I could not read behind his dark shades, but the vibes turned negative. He looked at me from behind his dark shades and then looked at Captain Hanafy and burst into laughter, a laughter that still rings in my ears until today.

"Are you kidding me? How can you bring me a fat boy like this to play in the professional team? Get him out of here."

Everyone joined him laughing at me. Mourad shooed me away with his hand like a fly before I had a chance to even blink. Blood rushed to my head. My cheeks burnt in the heat. My body froze and I felt I was going to faint. I wanted to disappear off the face of earth.

After he swatted the fat fly away, he shifted his attention to the boy who stood next to me, showering him with the smiles and nods he had just deprived me from. Saying that I felt ashamed is an understatement. I felt much worse than that. I was so shaken by the rejection, rendered speechless. Karim and the other players who were selected to the professional team were already in the court shooting hoops. Karim saw me walk away and continued his training, and as usual, he neither cared I was kicked out nor how I felt about it.

*

AFTER THE TRYOUTS

Numbed with shock, both emotionally and mentally, I picked up my training bag. With a heart heavier than my 125kg body weight, I carried my humiliation on my shoulder along with my bag, dragged my feet and walked away, wishing my heart would stop right there.

Despite my blurry vision and aching heart, I fought to hold back the tears. In a span of half an hour, my life flipped upside down. The pain and anger inside me were overwhelming. On the street, walking back to my house, the bitter taste of bile in my mouth nauseated me. I almost threw up. I walked like a zombie. My feet and mind were on autopilot, turned at the right intersections, stopped at the red lights, or not. I have no recollection of how I reached my destination, walked into the building and climbed up the flight of stairs to our apartment on the first floor.

The voices of the actors in the soap opera blaring from the TV in my mother's bedroom brought me back from my trance. Not in the mood for any interaction, I hurried to my room and closed the door behind me. I threw the training bag on the floor, laid in bed and gazed at the ceiling. With two hours before sunset, the room was bright. A ray of sunshine illuminated the face of Batman, perched in a poster on the wall in front of the bed. My superhero. I wondered if he too made fun of me.

In the safety of my room, my dark hole, the numbness melted away and emotions crept back inside me. The levee broke, and I cried. Tears flooded down my face. My mouth got very dry, I grabbed the bottle of water out of my training bag and gulped it to the last drop. I felt dizzy and weak. My breathing increased, my heart pounded and I broke into a sweat. My hands turned cold, my whole body shivered. As my sobbing continued, I felt the energy in my body depleting.

I laid there in frustrated rage, overwhelmed with anger and disappointment, at myself and the world. At that moment, I hated myself for my vulnerability and for my victimhood. On the one hand, I secretly believed I had a better chance than Karim, than most of the boys who were selected for the professional team. Taller, more focused and with higher shooting skills than most of them, I just needed a chance to prove my talent. On the other hand, part of me knew it was too good to be true. Captain Mourad woke me up from a dream I hoped would be mine, but never really belonged to me. With more tears shed, I scolded myself for believing I could actually make it to the professional team, for daring to dream.

The fact of the matter is I would never fit in basketball

or in any other sport. I never did and I never would. Mourad hadn't just rejected me. I was rejected even before he saw me. I was rejected at birth by a society intolerant to obese children. I was rejected when children bullied me in school and teachers did not care. I blamed myself for believing this time it would be different.

Since childhood, my mother forced me to play sports. I hated the sports she enrolled me in. She forced me to play football. I hated football. The coach also hated me for joining the team. More of a liability than a team member, he simply did not want me there, but he could not kick me out. For the junior teams, all kids were admitted, unless they had a health problem or a medical condition. Obesity is not a medical condition, just a nuisance. In the field, the children ran with the ball and I could not run, so no one passed the ball to me. The coach called me Fatso and mocked me in front of the other children. "Either you lose weight or you will be the goalkeeper," he repeated every training session. And he kept his promise. During most training sessions, I either sat on the bench or he forced me to protect the net, which in my case, the team players were more amused to hit me with the ball than to score.

I hated sports. I hated football with all my heart.

A knock on the door, and my mother's voice came from the

other side asking if I wanted dinner. "Yes," I responded. She did not ask anything else, and I did not volunteer to explain my day to her.

Already dark outside, I turned the light on and sat in bed with a plate of sandwiches by my side. I grabbed a video game from the bookshelf on my left where I kept my collection, put the volume down and pretended to be studying for the English class I enrolled in during the summer. I played video games until the early morning hours. I had morning classes at the British Council, and I knew if I did not get some rest, I wouldn't be able to make it to class. Despite my exhaustion, I did not want to sleep because I knew what would happen if I tried to.

When the events of the day finally took a toll on me, I turned the PlayStation off and closed my eyes. And as if someone turned a valve on, tears flooded from my eyes. I covered my face with my pillow, and cried myself to sleep. I did not want anyone to hear me crying. Other than Batman, I succeeded over the years to hide my feelings from my family, and not to cry in front of them. My pillow concealed my sobs. The tears Batman watched me shed over the years were enough to bloom some arid desert.

The following few days were business as usual. I met my parents casually in the hallways or in the kitchen. We often crossed paths in the living room too, but not long enough for them to notice my dilemma. I lost interest in playing basketball, but I went to classes at my regular hours. After classes I wandered the streets, alone. I resisted the temptation to go to the club to watch my peers playing basketball, embarrassed to be seen by any of them. When I returned back to my hole, my sanctuary, I studied, played video games and cried myself to sleep.

By the fourth day, I could not keep it inside me anymore. Whatever the consequences were, I was ready to spill it all out. Out of my bedroom, I followed the infusion of mouth watering aromas wafting from the kitchen. They led me to where my mother stood by the stove stirring the sizzling contents in a frying pan. Commercials played on the little kitchen TV. She gave me one of her enchanting smiles, the ones that glowed her face when in a good mood. She asked me if I was ready for breakfast.

I nodded; ready for more than just breakfast and I hated myself knowing that my confession would ruin her cheerful mood.

"Do you want me to prepare you an omelet?"

I shook my head. I opened the fridge and got out the cheese, stuffed many slices between the bread, many more slices than I should, and tossed them in the toaster oven. I love melted cheese in crispy bread. My mother turned on the percolator and added a spoonful of Nescafe inside my mug. She lowered the heat under the pan and started chopping some ripe tomatoes.

The toaster oven dinged and I removed the golden sandwich, with the cheese melted to perfection, and sighed. My mother's attention had already shifted to the morning show on TV.

"Mom, the coach kicked me out of the team."

She looked at me in confusion, "What? What coach? What team?"

Clueless about my basketball training or my interest to join the professional team, my statement caught her by surprise. She didn't even know I played basketball. She knew I trained occasionally, but as a hobby on my time off school, not that I had been in the junior team for three years.

Her concern about my education was the reason I played basketball behind her back. She only cared about my school work and studies. She did not encourage me to participate in any out-of-school activities or hobbies that might distract me from school work, sports included, if training sessions were offered during the school year. She wanted me to focus on my studies and to excel in school, to become the top in everything related to my education, as if to compensate my body with my brain. Because she believed that training would interrupt my studies, I did not mention it to her. During the school year, I pretended I had private lessons, but went to training instead. My father knew that I trained and let me.

My mother's jaw dropped and she gasped as I recounted to her the events of that fateful day, and how Mourad kicked me out and humiliated me in front of the team. She overcame her shock quickly, found her speech and scolded me so hard. She was both angry at me and for me. I saw the pain in her eyes, I knew it by heart. I had seen it before, more times than I can remember, or want to remember. Her pain for me was the main reason I stopped telling her what went on in my life.

She turned the stove off. Propelled with anger and frustration, she charged to my dad, taking it all out on him. She insisted he meets with Mourad to find out why he kicked me out of the team. Despite the obvious reason he spelled out in front of everybody, deep in her heart she wished the reason had nothing to do with my obesity.

I resisted going back, but my father convinced me that we should go. He, too, had hopes there might be another reason. Reluctantly, I returned to the scene of the crime. Nothing had changed in the three days of my absence; still chaotic, loud, animated, lively and fun. Mourad stood in the court looking like Darth Vader in his black coat. I hated his sight. The sounds of the balls dribbling, my former teammates shouting and the whistles blowing made my heart ache. I longed to be among them.

Karim ran back and forth with the ball. Even though I was hard to miss, he pretended he did not see me.

I stood next to my father by the sideline. We waited until the game ended to get a chance to talk with Darth Vader. My father introduced himself and asked him why he excluded me from the team.

Darth Vader had the response ready at the tip of his tongue, "Look at your son, don't you see how he looks?" He waved his arms in the air nonchalantly and walked away.

The hurtful words hit my father hard, like a punch in the face. He swallowed his pride and did not respond, could not respond, actually. With a light pat on my shoulder, we walked away in silence. In any American movie, the scene would end with the stadium lights turned out, but not this one. This was not a scene in a movie, but my true reality. I was embarrassed to cry in front of my father and the lump in my throat swelled, choking me. He did not miss my audible sniffles, but pretended he did not hear them.

Not the typical emotional man, my father could not empathize with me. "Son, there is nothing more we could do." My father's calculated tone rang in my ears. "Be a man. Toughen up and move on."

That was my father's way to show his solidarity with me. I could not hold my tears any longer and burst out crying. I dragged my feet next to him in silence, never felt lonelier in my life, in my teen life at least, as my childhood was nothing but loneliness. I wish I could have followed my father's advice and let it go. Unfortunately, I have never managed to get over this incident. The day Mourad kicked me out of the team had forever been engraved in my memory. It haunts me occasionally, until today, especially on days when I mess up my eating plan or have a bad exercise day. I have seen worse days in my childhood that I also remember on bad days. The incident with Mourad ended my basketball career. I never played or watched a game of basketball in my life since then. Until today, I cannot get myself to like it again.

Karim did not come to see me after the incident. He really did not care. He continued with his training, and we never talked about it when we ran into each other. In our childhood and during adolescence, we had a rough friendship, toxic at times. I believed he liked me, but he was also ashamed of me. Who wants to have an obese friend or be seen with one? At least not in public.

In a judgmental society, you are as cool as your friends and as those you hang out with. There is no tolerance for anyone who does not fit the social molds for coolness. I was a liability and an embarrassment to anyone who associated "himself" to me.

I did not write "herself" too, because of course other than my mother and sister, there was never another "she" and "her" in my life, until many years later. That did not go well either!

As a result, I had no one to share my feelings with. My brother, my only friend, would have been the person who could have comforted me, but he had already got married and moved out. I buried my feelings inside and continued on with my life. I have been living with the pain of that day until today. We all carry invisible scars that many do not know anything about. These scars have influenced and shaped us one way or another. It is not an exaggeration to say my expulsion from the basketball team is one of my invisible scars.

I retreated back to my dark hole, the one I had been living in all my life and was destined to live in for more years to come. No one would notice my absence, miss me or even remember me, if my name was ever mentioned. I would become invisible again, like my scars. In my dark hole, my only two faithful and loyal companions would not abandon me. Food and video games would cheer me up. They never failed me before.

Despite the trauma and emotional scars this incident left me with, regretfully, it was not the worst thing that had happened to me. My life up to that point has been nothing but misfortunate incidents, horrific at times, and it continued to be for a long time thereafter.

I AM NOT FAT

*

YEARS FROM HELL

A chubby baby is cute, until he's not – a baby, that is. I am my mother's first child and my father's third. My half-brother is 20 years older than me. My half-sister is 15 years older. They lost their mother to cancer at a young age and my mother raised them up.

Born to a loving mother, I was and still am the apple of her eye, the light of her life. She loved me unconditionally from the moment she gave birth to me, and fed me accordingly. Growing up in cultures where feasting is associated with its celebrations, food becomes part of people's lives, and often an obsession too. Egypt is not an exception. On the contrary, food is associated with everything we do. We meet when we are happy or sad and eat. And for every occasion, religious or otherwise, we have its traditional food. Family and friends gather and celebrate over recipes passed down over generations, some as old as ancient Egypt. In our home, we had an abundance of food, and fattening up a toddler, *"me"*, was not hard.

Cute chubby babies eventually lose their chub rolls as they grow, usually by the time they are ready for preschool. I did not. My chub rolls kept getting chubbier, the normal outcome when the calories I consumed exceeded the energy I burnt. At the age of 3 or 4, I did not know what calories meant, I wouldn't have understood what they are if someone mentioned the word to me, and of course I did not know calories counted – literally. And neither did my mother.

I do not blame my mother entirely for becoming an obese child, who grew up to become an obese adult. I do not blame her for many reasons, first and foremost, she overfed me out of love. Let's not blame our parents for everything wrong that happens in our lives. Secondly, motherhood does not come with a manual. When a child is crying from hunger, a mother would not deprive him from food, no matter what the outcome is. And that is what my mother did. There were other ways she could have handled it, but to the best of her knowledge, she was doing the right thing.

The most important reason I do not blame her is because I came to understand later in life that food is addictive. Simply put, I am a food addict. There is no shame here to admit it. Being a food addict is not her fault. People are just born with addictive personalities.

On the contrary, recognizing, admitting, and talking about the problem openly is the first step to solve it. Addiction to food is a fact of life I have to live with. During my journey with gaining and losing weight, I learned that addiction is a disease – an incurable one as a matter of fact. There are no explanations for why some people are born with addictive personalities and some are not. A normal child living with my mother wouldn't have gained the weight I did, because a child with a non-addictive personality would not have consumed the amount of food offered to me. A child with a non-addictive personality would not have used food for emotional comfort. A child with a non-addictive personality would not have second and third servings when he is full. A child with a non-addictive personality would eat only when he's hungry. A child with a non-addictive personality would stop eating when he is full, not when the heaps of food in front of him disappear.

A child with a non-addictive personality is not who I am.

While we cannot blame parents for their children's addictive personalities, they are still responsible for the quality of food their children consume. What parents feed their children, both in their stomachs and minds, in their first formative years, defines the pattern they would follow in life. Thus, it is important that parents should aspire to lead a healthy lifestyle, and teach that to their children too. Parents should not only feed the children healthy food that would not fatten them up, but also teach them the right eating habits. This, I would like to emphasize to new parents as well as to parents of obese children, there are always ways to right the wrongdoings.

In photographs from my kindergarten years, I was already an obese child for my age, but not yet a *freak* as people started calling me when I got older. My oversize body disabled me from leading a normal childhood. Back then, I did not understand why. Incompatible to children my age in the activities I participated in, I could not run like them. I could not ride a bike or even sit on a swing, since my weight exceeded the maximum allowance. Nonetheless, I was not aware yet of my body image, the social impact of obesity or that I was different. Children in kindergarten are more innocent, forgiving, tolerant of the others – traits that eventually fade as they get older.

Once I started school, it was a whole new game. I discovered the realities of life, or its nightmares, to be precise. I discovered the meaning of intolerance and bullying. I became the embodiment of a bullied child. Simply put, I became everybody's punching bag; classmates, teachers, relatives. Behind my back and in my face, neighbors, strangers in the streets and anyone who crossed my miserable path, had something unkind to say to me, and about me.

Bullying started in first grade and it came in all forms, physical, emotional and verbal. When the coolest boys in class made fun of me, everyone followed because laughing at the cool boys' jokes made them cool too.

No one wanted to be associated with me, so even those

who empathized with me, they also took part in humiliating and tormenting me. My classmates avoided me. They avoided hanging out with me, playing with me, or even talking to me entirely if they had the choice. Their choice was usually not in my favor. They kept their distance, as if I suffered from a contagious disease, a leper. At break time, I sat alone. I played alone. I ate alone. I watched life happening in front of me, a life I yearned to join, yet expelled from, because of my weight. I am still perplexed at how kids at such a young age harbor so much unkindness and cruelty, and have no shame expressing it, and even acting upon it.

Six-years-old children are in constant motion. With limited mobility, my classmates excluded me from their games, which at that age, most games required running, sprinting, climbing walls and trees. Activities I could neither participate in nor even remotely fantasize. It shouldn't be a surprise that no one wanted to sit with me when they had an exciting life going on for them.

I accepted being a loner and adapted to loneliness, but even minding my business and staying out of their way did not appeal to some of my classmates. I do not remember how the bullying started, but it seemed the more I withdrew to myself, the more they targeted me. I believe bullies are angry children, and bullying gives them pleasure and superiority. It feeds their egos. They circle the vulnerable and the weak and they dump their anger on them. They bully to substitute an emotional deficiency.

In school, I was physically violated for the first time in first grade. A classmate approached me during break time and for no other reason than because he wanted to, he shoved me, "Fatso, go sit in the classroom. I do not want to see you in the playground." Until today, I cannot comprehend what triggered such behavior in a six-years-old.

Life got worse in second grade, the year from hell is how I describe it. Second grade was the year that forever scarred me. Forever burnt in my memory, I remember it vividly. To date, I believe it was the worst year ever in my life – or maybe then abuse was still a novelty, and from there on it eventually became part of my life I learned to cope with – not that I had a choice.

In second grade, by the end of the first week in school, the class had divided into gangs, where members of each clustered together. Of course, I belonged to none. No one ever invited me to join his gang.

One day on the playground, some gangs fought together. As I stood watching, a gang leader approached me. "You are the tallest and fattest boy in class," he said, "we need your help." He ordered me to sit on top of a rival gang leader who had fallen on the ground, and was being kicked and stomped. I refused and before I could get out of his way, his gang circled me like hyenas and shoved me towards the fallen boy. They kicked me and pushed me. I fell on top of him. Everybody laughed, at me and at the boy under my weight, humiliated in front of his gang. I knew there and then, there would be blood.

The fallen gang leader pulled his body off the ground, dusty and soiled, and as he limped away he gave me the scariest look a six-years-old could give. He looked me in the eyes, spitted dirt and seethed, "I'll show you."

And he did.

Since that day, he had an ongoing vendetta with me that he settled daily. He dumped his anger and frustration on me because he could not beat the others, so he beat and humiliated me instead. He felt good punching me. He felt a winner abusing me. Bullying me salvaged his self-image and pride in front of his gang members.

I would not be exaggerating to say that he beat me every single day during this school year. Beating me was the kindest thing he did to me. On one occasion, he shoved me into the bathroom and forced me into a stall where he had just done his business, and forced me to grab his poop out of the toilet.

When I refused, he kicked me so hard with much venom. Seeing me holding his poop brought so much sickening pleasure on his face. His gang members had already surrounded us and watched in amusement as their hero restored their faith in him. They all took turns punching and kicking me. My body was sore and I had to hide my blue bruises from my mother for more than a week.

Boys often circled me and stuffed sand down my shirt; of course, I could not run fast enough from them to hide. In brief, I became their fun project.

I was mortified throughout second grade and completely helpless. When I complained to the teachers, no one stood up for me. No one took action to stop the bullying. The teachers did not bully me in the sense that they made fun of my weight, but I blame them for my sufferings and miseries. By being passive, they were accomplices. They may have not held the trigger, but they were there watching the crime without lifting a hand to stop it. Being passive, they might as well have joined the long queues of bullies who were after me.

No matter how much I complained to the teachers, no one really cared.

"It is okay. They did not mean to," was the answer I repeatedly heard from the class teachers. Their responses and reactions appalled me because these bullies intentionally abused me. Nothing was an accident.

While everything happened in front of their eyes, the teachers did not try to protect me either. They could have easily done that by allowing me to spend my break time in the teachers' room. I pleaded, I cried and I begged them to allow me to spend my break time there – I repeatedly told them I did not want to go to the playground. I did not want to play with anyone. Boys did not beat me in the teachers' room, but they wouldn't listen to me. The teachers forced me out of their room, the only sanctuary I had in school. They did not believe me. They said they were sick of our stupid games. They did not care what the children did or did not do. Teaching was just a job that provided them with an income, nothing more.

And of course, the boys knew my hiding place, and guess what? Whenever I had a chance to sneak in and hide inside the teachers' room during recess, they waited for me outside and beat me up the minute I stepped out. Hello teachers.

On the one occasion a teacher witnessed the boys beating me up, she scolded them, and then she turned and scolded me too, as if it was my fault. In this sense, I hold the teachers responsible for the torment and pain I endured in silence. I do not know until today how I survived these hard times.

What antagonized me the most, was that every time I came back to my mother soiled, bruised, bloody and disheveled, and told her what had happened to me, she too, scolded and beat me up. She beat me up for allowing the boys to bully me and for not standing up to them. It was a double whammy for me, caught between the rock and the hard place.

"Do not let them do that to you," she told me repeatedly. Not that I lacked courage to fight or hit back, I was bigger in size than all of them, but I really did not want to beat up anyone. I did not want to be violent or aggressive with them. I did not want to end up like them.

"You are big and tall. How could you not beat them back?"

When I look back, I believe deep down I did not want to beat them up because I did not want them to be angry or upset with me. That is how desperate I was for love and acceptance.

When I complained or cried to my mother, she whacked me, and I learned then to hide from her what happened in my life. As I got older, I realized that her intentions were not to hurt me, but rather to toughen me up. She took out on me the anger she had at them for what they did to me. She visited the school twice or maybe three times and talked to the teachers and principal, to no avail. From my end, I stopped complaining to her as it only brought her pain.

My father spent most of his time at work, and we did not have a close relationship to start with, so I hardly told him any of my problems, or anything else – per se. I loved my sister, and she loved me back, but we weren't close to each other, not at all, even though she lived one room away from me. She was and still a very sweet person, but we had different mentalities, even back then.

I found solace and comfort with my brother. In my distress or despair, I sought him. In spite of the 20 years' difference in age between us, he was the closest to me and my best friend. He listened to me and comforted me, in his own way. He taught me video games and we played them together. Every Friday he took me to buy a new game. Of all the people in my life, I only enjoyed my brother's company.

I hated school. I hated school beyond words can describe, and I did not want to go because I knew how my days would end up. I found excuses to skip school. Every day I pretended I was sick. Unfortunately, it did not work all the time. By the end of the school year, my mother could not tolerate what I had to endure every day, coming home beaten, abused, injured and crying. So, when a relative recommended another school with better academic records, my mother grabbed the opportunity. We visited the new school and she liked it immediately. I bet she would have liked it no matter what. Deep inside, she too had had enough of what went on in my life.

No one was more relieved to hear the news than I did. I

was ready for a new beginning. When the new school started, I was ready for a fresh start. It turned out to be just wishful thinking.

A NEW SCHOOL. A NEW BEGINNING, OR NOT

The school bell rings and revives my classmates, as if pumping blood into their veins. They erupt in euphoric jubilation; their early yawns of boredom at the mathematics equations scribbled on the blackboard are replaced with cheers. With this rebirth of energy, they dash out of the classroom like an avalanche, no one paying attention to the teacher who stands there, his lips moving, but his voice muffled by the noise.

Excitement is contagious. The voices grow louder as students roar and stomp down the stairs in an organized chaos, pushing and shoving their way like a herd of wild beasts, racing to freedom. PE class is the second-best thing in school after break time. It is a legitimate freedom to exercise, jump, run around, or perhaps play a game of football, depending on the mood of the PE teacher. Not that I care for any, yet skipping a class is every fifth grader dream.

My classmates race to the locker room, the first out in the field will enjoy extra precious minutes of playtime. The PE teacher stands by the entrance, blocks our way. We gather in front of and around him. As the noise escalates, he blows his whistle. "Boys, class is cancelled today," he announces.

He catches our attention. The crowd gasps inquisitively and everyone talks in the same breath, out of control. He blows another long piercing whistle.

"There is a medical checkup today. You all have to go to the clinic. Go ahead. I will follow you there."

"A medical what?"

Eyes-roll and shoulders shrug, and along with the looks of disappointment for cancelling the class, there were many curious looks trying to understand what was going on.

"What is a medical checkup?" students ask curiously.

"The nurse will check your blood pressure and weight."

"What?"

"Why?"

I remember that day vividly, burnt in my memory among many similar ones. It happened early in the school year. No one in class understood what a medical checkup is, its purpose or significance, if any. It must have been a spur-of-the-moment decision by someone. Parents were not notified and no one asked for their permission. The school just did it. Until today, I have no idea why they conducted it, who asked for it or why, and where they kept the results. Most importantly, throughout my years in school, and until I graduated from high school, it never happened again.

The PE teacher blows more whistles. They echo in our ears and the students disperse. They run in different directions, none leading to the clinic. The energy saved for the PE class transforms to roars of anger, excitement and perhaps curiosity, all mixed together. I arrive at the clinic before the others who linger in the corridors and hallways, in no hurry to reach their destination. Not that I was anxious to get there, but being an outcast, I had no reason to delay, for no one hangs out or plays with me.

Two students beat me there, though. Inside the clinic, the school nurse sits at her desk with a stethoscope around her neck. A closed file lays in front of her, with a glass of hot steaming tea and a packet of biscuits next to it. A poster of the digestive system hangs above her head. The air smells of this distinctive disinfectant they use in hospitals. Our appearance in the doorway interrupts her peace, and breakfast. She gives us a stern look and purses her lips.

"Stand in line," she says, nonchalantly.

She points to a scale with a telescoping height measuring rod, then pulls out a biscuit from the packet and stuffs it in her mouth. She mutters under her breath and gazes the other direction, where the poster of the respiratory system hangs above the black treatment table that looks like a massage table. When she clears her mouth from the biscuit, she blows on the tea and slurps it. The vapor fogs her glasses, but just for a moment.

"What is this about?" the student in front of me asks. I do not know his name. He is also a fifth grader, but in another class. We meet in PE classes.

"I do not know," she shrugs and pulls out a pen from the pocket of her white coat. She opens the file in front of her, stares at the papers inside it, and taps the pen on the desk.

We stand by the scale where she pointed. As more students drizzle in, she stuffs another biscuit in her mouth and puts the packet inside the drawer. Breakfast time is over. With some luck, she may finish the tea before the PE teacher arrives.

She sits up straight, adjusts the veil on her head and taps the pen harder, to remind us to stay quiet, but to no avail.

"Stand in line," she tells everyone who walks in. She knows us all, maybe not by name, but she certainly recognizes our faces. And in my case, my body too. My size is recognizable a mile away.

I stand third in line behind a chubby boy, but I was much bigger, by far. The queue behind me gets long and snakes out of the door and into the corridor. A whistle echoes and voices calm down.

The PE teacher appears in the doorway. His sneakers

squeak on the tile floor. The nurse gulps the hot tea to the last drop. I wonder how she did not burn her mouth or throat. She stands up, hands the teacher the file and the pen. From a small cabinet in the corner located under charts of what we eat, she grabs a blood pressure monitor.

The first boy in line gives his name and class. The nurse measures his blood pressure, height and weight. She reads the numbers out to the PE teacher and he writes them down in the file. My stomach clenches as I watch. I focus on a poster of the body muscles, realizing I had none.

When it is my turn, she tightens the cuff of the blood pressure monitor around my upper arm, places the stethoscope on my vein and inflates the cuff, until my arm hurts, and then she decreases the pressure. I would have been more interested to follow the process; had I not been focused on what would happen next. She reads my blood pressure to the PE teacher. He writes it down. I could not tell from his expression whether it is a good number or a bad one.

She stands next to the scale and asks me to step on it. I look at it, at her and shake my head. My cheeks burn from the heat of embarrassment. Behind me, the curious eyes of the fifth-grade students are wide open, waiting in anticipation to find out the number. I was the fattest child in the class, perhaps the fattest in the school too.

"You have to," she interrupts my thought.

"I do not want to."

The nurse takes a deep breath, sighs impatiently as she exchanges looks with the PE teacher.

I am at the verge of tears. I bite my lips to control myself from crying. There is no way out. I had to do as I was told. We can go on forever, but the only thing I will accomplish is attract more attention.

I take a deep breath, gather my courage and step on the scale, my knees wobble as I whisper to her, beg her not to read the number out loud.

I see the number. The nurse gasps in shock, "This cannot be," she bursts out and looks at the PE teacher. I feel the sweat beads gather on my forehead and on my burning cheeks. I squeeze my eyes to fight the tears.

The children behind watch the show as it unfolds. No one interrupts, no one talks.

"Step down and try again," the nurse says.

Same reading.

The nurse shakes her head in disbelief. "The scale is malfunctioning," she tells the PE teacher.

The PE teacher approaches. I get off the scale. He leans over and adjusts something, some dials, who knows, and asks me to step on it again. Amid the commotion their voices grow louder.

"He's 90 kg. There is nothing wrong with the scale," barks the PE teacher.

"90 kg! No way. He's just 11," the nurse screams out in shock.

Everyone hears her voice, loud and clear. The students repeat it like an echo, just to make sure no one misses it.

I feel embarrassed, broken. I want to disappear from the face of earth.

Behind me I first hear gasps, muffled voices, whispers, giggles and then laughter, loud, wicked and vicious. From the nurse room, the word spreads like forest fires throughout the school. Now everyone knows how much I weigh. Thanks to the chattery news reporters, my classmates.

The memory of the medical check-up day gives me nightmares until now. The scale actually read 90.5 kg. I saw it with my eyes. This number is also burnt in my memory. The students were left in shock. The number certainly looked massive when compared to their weights. With a basic mathematics formula, they found out I weighed almost double their sizes. For the rest of that school year I became known as the boy who weighed 90 kg. The boy who almost broke the scale.

It was a hellish year, to say the least. A year filled with

sarcasm and humiliation. They yelled behind me, and even in my face with no shame or guilt, "Hey 90 kilos."

It became my name, label and description.

I did not tell my mother.

Fifth grade was also a turning point in my life, a wakeup call. I started to realize the importance of social appearance. For the first time, I became self-aware of how I looked. By then, bullying had become more verbal than physical. Bullies had also discovered that sharp tongues are effective weapons too. They did not have to waste their energy to beat me up if they can inflict pain on me with their comments and hurtful words. Not that they stopped beating me up entirely, it just happened less frequently, and not with the same force or intensity. They still pushed me around, shoved me against a wall, threw water, bottles and cans at me as I walked by. Once, someone aimed a half-full can at my head and injured me. Often they surrounded me, shoved me around until I fell and they laughed. I cannot really pinpoint what goes through the mind of bullies, but whatever it was, they found it amusing. On one occasion, I slipped and lost my consciousness on the way down. I blacked out on the ground. When I recovered my consciousness, the teacher scolded me along with the bullies, as if it was my fault.

They bullied me the entire school year for no reason – just because I was different. Because I was big. Because I looked scary.

*

Obesity is a kind of a mental illness. It is a vicious cycle, a closed disease, a mental box. I call it a loop. I eat because I am upset. I am upset because I am fat. And because I am fat, people bully me and bad things happen to me in my life. Things that are out of my control. Things I do not want to happen, or wish to happen, but they happen anyway, because of how I look. I find nothing to compensate for the pain and the trauma I am in except food and eating. Food was my companion, my friend, my comfort. I ate because my feelings were hurt. I ate because I was angry. I was a very angry child. Food made me less angry, despite not fixing the problem that caused my anger in the first place. This is the loop I am referring to.

The problem is also with people, their attitudes, behaviors and reactions toward anyone who's slightly different than them. I am not talking here about just obesity, but any kind of difference. Obese, skinny, short, tall, with mental or physical challenges; if you do not fit in the traditionally accepted social mold, they will bully you, exclude you from their circle and reject you, for something that is 99 percent of the time not your fault, or you have control over it. Period. That bothered me the most.

I did not choose the way I looked. I did not choose the card life handed me. I did not even choose my genes. Until today, I hate my genes. I do not blame my parents for them. It is not their fault either. Understanding that, however, does not make the frustration go away every time I crave food because something upset me or angered me.

I wish to live a normal life. I wish I could stop thinking about food, but I can't. I wish I can only eat when I am hungry, like normal people do. But that is not the case. I have to watch everything I eat. I have to diet, exercise, and live with hunger pangs, day in and day out, to lose weight, or stay in shape to look good, to become socially acceptable. It is a never-ending struggle, yet people do not understand that – people do not have empathy for it. People do not care about you, they really do not! They are experts at labeling and judging you, though.

In their closed minds, many believe obese people have no willpower or self-discipline. They think of obese people as procrastinators who do not want to close their mouths and watch the fat melting away. They draw their images in their minds as weak individuals with no determination to go through the pain it takes to lose weight. Regretfully, they judge them from the perspective of normality. Perhaps overweight normal people are weak and lack willpower, determination and self-discipline; cannot keep their mouths closed to endure the pain it takes to lose weight. However, for food addicts, it is a different game. For food addicts, it is a battle, a war; a never-ending war, as a matter of fact. It ends when one dies. It is as simple as that.

Food addiction is the hardest of addictions to quit. It is even harder than drug addiction. Just think for a moment here. People do not need drugs to survive. Recovered drug addicts can live without using drugs, but can people survive without food? Food addicts have to stop eating to lose weight, yet they still have to taste the substance of their addiction to survive.

However, there is always hope. I believe deep down we, obese people, were cursed by a blessing in disguise. We were born to be different. Why keep trying to fit in when we can actually stand out so easily.

Let me explain why we develop an emotional connection with food. In his book, The Power of Habits – which literally changed my life - Charles Duhigg explains that there are a group of subcortical nuclei called basal ganglia, located deep inside our brains and are responsible for our automation system. This includes walking, running, talking, driving. They are automated body functions that do not require our conscious awareness. However, when we build a habit, basal ganglia start to take control of it until it too becomes automated. Therefore, we find ourselves eating without even realizing it!

There is a secret that marketers use in their advertisements called the habit loop. The habit loop consists of three parts; the cue, the routine and the reward. The cue triggers the habit. For example, when you wake up in the morning and you see the sunshine you crave coffee, so you drink coffee. The cue is waking up and seeing the sun, it is automated. The routine is the habit itself, drinking coffee every morning. Then comes the reward. Drinking coffee makes you happy and refreshed because it stimulates the release of dopamine, the hormone of happiness. This chemical spikes when you are "feeling good" because you are experiencing and enjoying pleasurable events.

Now let me explain how food is used in the same concept. The brain records the activities that produce dopamine and tends to resort to them when we are sad, bored, or filled with negative emotions. That is the reason why anything can be addictive, including food. When an obese person is bullied, humiliated or mocked, the brain see the cue which in this case is sadness and frustration. The obese person immediately craves for food because the brain chooses the easiest and fastest way to produce dopamine, which is eating, and that is called emotional eating. Do not blame the brain. It is trying to make us happy.

I was trapped in this loop.

*

After the medical checkup in fifth grade, some genius in school, as if discovered a new revelation, suggested that to lose weight, I had to stop eating. My classmates took it upon themselves to assure I did not eat during break time. They started stealing my lunch. Well, they actually did not steal it behind my back, they forced me to surrender it, unwillingly. They waited for me as I came out of class, ganged around me and snatched my lunchbox. They were many, and they were mean and vicious. They scared and humiliated me. I gave them my food.

I did not tell my mother they stole my food, but I asked her to prepare me more, to double whatever she filled my lunchbox with. She did not question my request, she simply thought I was always hungry. In school, I hid half the food my mother prepared for me. I kept it as reserve, to dig out of my bag once they left me in peace, after they walked away with the contents of my lunchbox. I guess I was lucky. They never discovered I had extra food with me.

Life became intolerable in my second school. I resorted to my two companions; food and video games. During the school year, my mother confiscated the video games so I would focus on studying. I was left with nothing but food, the only relief that took my pain away. But with all the torment and suffering in school, I had reached a stage where not even food took away the pain and humiliation, and I asked my parents to move me to another school.

At this young age, I never saw moving from one school to another as running away from myself, but rather running away from my circumstances. Unfortunately, it took me a while to realize that the circumstances were me. In all the schools that I moved to, I was the one constant thing, the common factor in all the places and with all the people who rejected and avoided me. With the new move, I was adamant to become acceptable. I was determined to blend it.

*

THIRD TIME'S A CHARM

I arrived at my third school carrying a lot of baggage on my shoulders; sacks heavier than my heart, heavier than my weight, no pun intended. Sacks loaded with emotional pain, shame, torment, rejection, open wounds, anger, disappointment, desperation and loneliness, to mention a few. I had witnessed and suffered ugly experiences beyond the comprehension of a fifth grader. Regretfully, they had already shaped my formative years, scarred my soul and defined my future.

But as they say, every ending is a new beginning, and I embraced this saying wholeheartedly. Bidding farewell to my old school was the beginning of a new phase in my life. As a transfer student, despite the anxieties and misery I dragged along with me to the new school, yet with the anonymity of my past experiences and the meager knowledge of the world I acquired at that age, I decided to step over my shame and vulnerability and change my circumstances. I vowed I would not be a doormat or punching bag anymore. I would not be left behind, hide in a corner and lick my wounds. Evidently, I had no plans on how to restore my damaged self-esteem and violated dignity. Nonetheless, I was adamant to blend in and to become someone, whatever that takes.

I had also made up my mind to change my self-image. For this, I knew what to do. I was aware I needed to exercise regularly to lose weight. Cutting down on the quantity or quality of food I ate was non-negotiable, never even considered this option. I joined the basketball academy at the club. Despite my dislike for sports, I desperately wanted to change. Playing basketball was my contribution to my new beginning, my new goals, my new me. I also wanted to meet new people. Whatever it would have taken me to make friends, I would have done it.

I started at my new school as a blank slate. My obesity still invited sarcasm and humiliation. However, my new schoolmates were oblivious to my bullying history and emotional torment. It was up to me how I presented myself to them. Showing any weakness or vulnerability would have been similar to dumping blood in the ocean to attract sharks. I was determined to keep their sharp teeth away from me.

I came up with a strategy; become proactive rather than reactive. If I hang out with the coolest and most popular kids in school, I would be associated with them, and become accepted by everyone else. Over the years, I grew aware that the impression we give people is a reflection of how we portray and carry ourselves. Unfortunately, in my previous school, I got stuck in a mold impossible to break. With the perpetuation of bullying and humiliation, any attempt to alter the image I gave to my schoolmates was doomed to failure.

In the new school, I had the opportunity to pretend to be anyone I chose, to portray myself in any way I wanted. As a newcomer, I lingered and hovered around the cool kids and smiled at their jokes about me. No one stopped me from approaching them. I did not threaten their coolness or popularity. On the contrary, they needed me to enhance their coolness. You find me in buddy films. People like me are brought to movies to contrast the protagonists, as our differences accentuate their macho images. A tall handsome well-built character in a movie hangs out with a short, ugly and overweight buddy. Cool guys needed buddies like me to shine.

Hovering around them was easier than blending in though. The latter required more effort. I studied the cool guys, their moves, gestures, how they walked, laughed, talked, the expressions they used, the shows they watched, the music they listened to, the comics they read, the brand of clothes they wore. I frequented their after school hangouts. I inhaled everything they did, even the cigarettes they offered me. They smoked, I smoked. I copied just about everything they did. I imitated them. I molded my character after theirs. I became them. I became someone I did not recognize.

In a misfortunate incident in my school, I stumbled and

fell down the stairs. Not that it came as a surprise, but everyone laughed at me. My fall amused them. The new me did not shy away though. I used the fall to my advantage. I stood up and joined them laughing at me. They laughed even more. From that moment on, I became the clown of the class. The one they made fun of. I intentionally assumed this role to be accepted. I played the class fool to draw laughter. I invented foolish acts to amuse them, make them laugh, entertain them, just to be included in their circle. I have lived all my life on the edge and in the shadow, always watching from the outside like an intruder. When I finally got a chance to step inside the circle, I grabbed it. The new feeling of acceptance was warm and fuzzy. It did not matter how I got there and I had no intention to compromise, risk or give up what I have accomplished.

 I tried everything just to have friends and keep them. I became a people's pleaser. I bought their friendship with laughter, lent them my video games, bought them meals when we went out, and as an A student, I often helped them with schoolwork. At the end, I succeeded in having some companions. I cannot describe them as friends because even if I considered them so, I was just an acquaintance to them. They sought my company when they had nothing else to do or no one else to hang out with. I was their spare tire, their plan B or even C. No one understood me. No one cared about me. No one cared to know me. And honestly, I did not give a damn. I finally had boys my age to hang out with and that was all that mattered.

At the club, I became obsessed with basketball, especially after the club hired Coach Hanafy who took me under his wing and helped me improve my shooting skills. He saw in me what no one else saw. With the pass of time, I became keen to join the club's first team. And with every training day, I became more confident I would make it. I practiced every day, for three continuous years. My basketball skills improved, but I have to admit, even my fierce exercise did not drop my weight. I consumed more calories than I burned. The curse of junk food accompanied me for a long time in my life. The curse of my weight accompanied me to the basketball court all the way until the team qualification games. Because of my weight Coach Mourad kicked me out of the team.

I do not know what came to my mind after Mourad kicked me out of the team – that led me to parkour. I have liked parkour since I was a child. I cannot recall exactly when I became obsessed with it, but it was like a dream that grew with me. When I played video games, I was awed at how the characters flipped, slided, spinned, jumped and flew, and I fantasized about playing it. When my short-lived basketball career ended, my buried dream popped to the surface.

Whether it was my obsession with video games, Batman hanging on my wall urging me to become a hero myself, the desire to prove to everyone I can compete just like them, that my weight is not an obstacle, even if they saw it otherwise, or all of the above, I became determined to play parkour. I wanted to prove them all wrong.

Parkour was the straw that broke the camel's back.

*

PARKOUR: PURSUING A BURIED PASSION

Assassin's Creed was my favorite video game. I became obsessed with the game, the stories and characters. My favorite was Ezio Auditore da Firenze, the Italian master assassin, who plays the protagonist in the games set during the Italian Renaissance.

Of all the characters of Assassin's Creed, in my opinion, and I believe many who played the game will agree with me, Ezio is the most popular character. He came from an affluent noble family of bankers in Florence. He lived a privileged life until the age of 17, unaware of his father's underground ties with the Assassin Order. His pampered life changes after he witnesses the hanging of his father and brothers. He joins the ranks of the assassins to avenge their death. His quest takes him to Spain and the lands of the Ottoman empire. He reestablishes the Order of Assassins in Italy and becomes the Mentor of the Italian Brotherhood of Assassins.

The beauty of his character is in how it developed over time. He started just like one of us. A vulnerable young man, he was not bred to become a master assassin, but his circumstances led him to that path. He trained hard and we watched as he grew and transformed. He learned the fighting techniques from his friends and allies. His abilities and power unfolded in front of our eyes. I instantly clicked with Ezio.

A couple of years older than me when put to test, yet the way he handled and developed himself inspired, motivated, and most of all fascinated me. After my expulsion from basketball, I felt defeated. I lost interest in just about anything, other than food and video games. In the safety of my black hole, I spent countless hours with Ezio. He became my superhero.

With a body built to perfection by computer animation software, Ezio mastered the parkour moves. He swiftly flipped and vaulted in the air as he jumped from building to building. No obstacle challenged him. No barriers stopped him. He conquered both his physical and mental fears and rose in the ranks to become the best.

I wanted to become Ezio. It did not matter he lived in a fictional world and I lived in the real one. It did not matter he was slim and I obese, or he could run, climb the side of buildings, jump between rooftops or cross barriers, while I sat in bed and pressed some buttons. All I could think of, if Ezio could do it, I could do it. And there was only one way to become Ezio, play parkour.

Parkour fascinated me before I knew its name. It is not

really a sport, but rather a discipline, as it became known globally. Since its birth in the suburbs of Paris in the eighties by a handful of young guys who trained and played together, it developed and evolved over the years to become what it is today. Assassin's Creed video games were the first to heavily borrow parkour moves, and as the game swept the world by storm, playing parkour became every gamer's secret dream.

The parkour frenzy found its way to Egypt and I became adamant to play it. If you haven't played Assassin's Creed or are not familiar with parkour, in brief, it is a physical activity where players challenge obstacles in whatever environment they are in without using tools, equipment or assistance from others. The obstacles can be tall walls, rails, jumping from high buildings or jumping from one building to the other. It is about strength and speed. Thus, the challenge for the players is not only in overcoming these obstacles using their physical abilities alone, but also how they do it.

When it started, parkour was limited to moves borrowed from combat. But its founders did not start it as a regimented exercise. They set no rules or regulations to how it should be practiced. That invited players over the years to add, tweak, modify or invent new moves. The game became bound only by the imagination and creativity of its players. Whatever moves they imagined, they had the freedom to adopt; front and back flipping, vaulting, crawling, swinging, walking on rails, climbing walls, jumping barriers or jumping of them became part of its techniques, and we haven't seen the end of it yet.

Parkour is dynamic and it will keep evolving as long as people are playing it. With no restrictions, it is open to change and adaptability to meet every player's need and environment. We forget how amazing our bodies are or the amazing things our bodies can do, but parkour players remind us of that. Any new movement the players imagine, they push their limits and train themselves to do it.

To say parkour became my obsession is an understatement. I talked about nothing but parkour. It became like a flame burning inside me and occupied every minute of my waking hours. I daydreamed, wished and hoped for nothing but to play it. My life changed when one of my school friends broke the news to me that a group of young people had formed a team to play and teach parkour. They called themselves Parkour Egypt. He suggested we go and watch them in action.

"But you do not understand. I do not want to watch them. I want to play parkour," I explained to him.

He shook his head, "It is a sport for thin people."

As if I did not already know that. Just look at Ezio. He has not one gram of fat in his body.

"I can do it."

He rolled his eyes and walked away.

By then, my efforts and strategies to blend in and become accepted had finally paid off and I managed to make some friends at school. My social life slightly improved. Karim and two other friends shared my enthusiasm to visit the training grounds of Parkour Egypt and watch the guys flip in the air.

We visited **Sadeya** School located next to the University of Cairo. The school is the largest public school in Egypt and has courts and playgrounds for just about any sport. Members of Parkour Egypt trained there. Watching them in action was better than anything I had imagined. The interest of the two friends stopped there. But Karim, who had already been kicked out of basketball, decided to give it a try. Of course, he also did not take me seriously when I told him I wanted to play parkour.

Karim not believing in me was the least of my problems. I had obstacles and challenges even parkour buffs could not overcome. I am not talking here about my weight, but how to convince my mother to allow me to play.

My mother did not want to hear about anything that would distract me from school work or endanger my life. Parkour combined both of her fears. Playing parkour was out of the question. My mother reluctantly accepted after I pleaded and begged for weeks, and after I assured her that playing it will not affect my studies, and that I would be careful not to injure myself. I also promised her I will only play on weekends and school breaks; a promise I never kept.

Karim was not the only one who did not believe in my ability to play parkour, just about everyone else in the team did not either. They discouraged me from joining even before I signed up. My body size and shape did not convince them I could play. Of course, I was aware of my limitations. I knew I could not be like them, nonetheless, I insisted I will commit to it no matter what.

When I joined, I became the new attraction of the team. They were curious to watch me in action, watch me fall, watch me fail. They had doubts someone my size could flip. I had doubts myself, but I was ferociously determined to do it. Every training session, without exaggeration, they welcomed me with discouraging, demeaning and humiliating comments.

"You will not be able to flip, ever."

"How can someone your size play parkour?"

"Go lose weight and come back."

The more they antagonized me, the more I wanted to prove them all wrong. The more they humiliated me, the more determined I was to flip. Flipping became my utmost desire, and dream.

Parkour became my outlet. I could not wait for the

school day to end to go to training. In class, I daydreamed about it. I sat in class doodling Parkour Egypt logo in my notebooks, counting the hours until I can get there. That is how much I loved it.

I trained three days a week for three years. Saturdays, Mondays and Wednesdays. I did not miss a day of training. **I had my good training days and my bad ones.** The training sessions started with pushups and pullups for warm up. Then each session focused on one move, and we spent the entire time trying it out; front flip, back flip, rolling, obstacle jumping, monkey jumps, dash and speed vaults, and so on. We also trained several styles. My progress was slower in comparison to the others, but I was persistent. And despite my continuous exercise, **my weight remained the same.**

Karim on the other hand advanced quickly. During the first year, he learnt to front and back flip, and by the end of the year he joined the first team. It took me way longer than that to reach this level, but with persistence, I eventually learned front and back flips. Of course, landing on my feet was hard, with sharp pain shooting in my legs and knees, but I did it. I looked up to Karim, consulted him and he gave me feedback on my techniques. Despite my slow progress, he still never took me seriously.

I heard two guys talking over my head one day. One was a

newcomer to the team. "He's so fat. He cannot flip," said the new comer.

"I bet you he can, he will flip."

"No way," replied the newcomer in sarcasm.

Their comments challenged me, but I pretended I did not hear them and continued my training. When the chance came and I saw the newcomer looking in my direction, I flipped and landed on my feet. From the corner of my eyes, I saw the guy's jaw drop in awe. I smiled to myself. It was a moment of triumph. I proved them all wrong.

*

Let me tell you this. When you play parkour, you impress people. Even if they pretend otherwise, they elevate you to the ranks of the cool guys. Just think about it. How many people do you know jump rails, climb buildings and flip in the air on their way up? Also, when you play parkour, you brag about it and show off at every opportunity. The Dokki Shooting Club became the outlet where Karim and I showed off our new talents. Whenever we went there, which was quite often, we performed parkour moves to impress whoever happened to cross our path. And if the passerby were basketball players, we went the extra mile to impress them even more. Even then, Karim had not taken me seriously still.

Karim to a greater level maintained better relations with the basketball team than I. He was kicked out of the team for lack of discipline, causing troubles with other players and missing training. In their eyes, he was a rebel not an incompetent obese who crowded the court and slowed down the game; one they laughed at with no empathy when their coach humiliated him and kicked him out of the team.

After each flip in the air, I stopped to watch the look of awe on the faces of those who watched me. Their popping eyes and dropping jaws filled me with pride. A feeling I was neither familiar with nor accustomed to, yet I immensely enjoyed. That is how parkour changed my life. It boosted my self-confidence. It helped me overcome my insecurities and cope with many issues and challenges in my life; and I had an abundance of insecurities and issues to last me two lifetimes.

Many who are unfamiliar with parkour training believe the physical aspect of the game is the hardest. This is not correct. Mentally, parkour is equally challenging. To be able to perform the moves, the mind requires a different setting that can only be acquired by extreme focusing and concentration. Parkour is not just about what the body can do, but how to set your mind to put the self-preservation mode on hold, and override it to allow you to perform these moves.

When I focused and concentrated hard, I forgot about

anything else in my life. The world around me ceased to exist. I turned the power switch off and shut the world and its troubles down. When I played, the feelings of body shame were put on hold. I did not care how I looked in the eyes of others, either. All that consumed me was how to lift my legs off the ground, how to convince my body to soar. To just do it. When I flipped in the air, my body image faded away. I forgot about my weight and I became in full harmony with my surroundings. As if the moment froze and I moved in slow motion. Parkour was freedom. Liberation. I never experienced similar feelings before, or since then.

Even though it had less impact on improving my body shape, it helped me develop my mental skills and overcome my emotional problems. It helped me realize that this world is mine too and I have the right to be part of it, even though many believed I belonged on the sidelines. Overcoming the mental fear reflected on other angles in my life, like conquering my self-doubt and social dysfunction. It also bettered my self acceptance. In total, my awkwardness dwarfed as my skills improved.

All things considered, I felt good about myself. For the first time in my life my body weight was not an obstacle—well it was in a sense, but I considered the fact that I managed to overcome it a miracle in itself.

"Hey! Up for a game of Death Match this weekend?"

Hazem asked me one day at break time.

When you become a cool guy, because you play parkour, you are accepted by the even cooler guys in school. The ones you have always looked up to and emulated. These moments when they plan an outing and include you are priceless. At school, my efforts at becoming the class clown, the people pleaser, and their clone, finally paid off. The cool guys noticed me, accepted me. Not to mention how playing parkour impressed them and cemented my position in the gang. Certainly, they did not include me in their more intimate outings, but they welcomed me for the ones they needed a large group to play a game. I did not mind. I welcomed whatever invitation thrown my way.

"Omar's father is away and Omar managed to get his car," Hazem added.

When you play parkour, people look at you differently. I was no longer the guy who is out of breath, but someone who can actually compete with them. I felt good about myself. The invitation from Hazem, the coolest guy in school, to join them for a game of paintball thrilled me. I finally had friends.

My chest swelled with pride, "you bet."

*

THE ACCIDENT

In high school, paintball had just been introduced in Egypt, and playing it became every teenager's dream, including myself, of course. Playing a game of paintball emulated a real video game. The excitement and fun it brought to me was worth the trouble driving to Adrenaline Park, in October city. Not to mention saving my allowance for weeks to afford the game, and even lying to my mother about it.

My overprotective mother never let me go out with my friends, except if the outing involved a study group or a private lesson. She also allowed me to go to parkour training on my days off from school, after she made sure I finished my school assignments.

Growing up in an environment where everything was off limits, I learned early on to do things behind her back. Sorry mom. She gave me many reasons why I should not do this or that. I heard her reasons loud and clear, but she never convinced me. Reading between the lines, I understand she tried to shield me from abuse and bullying, in the only way she could, by preventing me from going out. She also wanted me to excel in school, to give her a reason to impress the family and friends who continuously stabbed her with their hurtful remarks about my weight. Nonetheless, her overprotection often suffocated me, and despite her watchful eyes, I managed to sneak out whenever I had the chance.

Paintball, the competitive team shooting sport is the brainchild of the two Americans, Hayes Noel, a stockbroker, and Charles Gaines, a journalist. In the game, players shoot gelatin balls at each other from special guns. The balls are filled with colored dye and break when they hit a target. Players are eliminated when they are hit by these balls. The winning team is the one that eliminates the players of their opponent team first.

Noel and Gains did not invent the idea though, as paintball guns were invented in the sixties and used by foresters to mark trees on challenging terrains. Farmers also used paintballs to mark their livestock. However, Noel and Gains utilized the idea of paintball, and with the help of a third friend they created the recreational sport known today. They formed a team of twelve men and played the first game of paintball in New Hampshire in 1981. Paintball is also used, in the US and many other countries, by the military and police forces for their training.

Paintball is all about adrenaline rush and heart pumping. It excited me as much as parkour, especially that some of my parkour skills came handy too. And to be asked to join the coolest guys in school for a game was the cherry on the pie. I would never have turned the invitation down, no matter what it cost me. I plotted for days to lay the foundation for the excuse to give my mother. She believed my story about the revision lesson the private tutor was giving at a friend's.

On a good day, Adrenaline Park is an hour drive away. We booked in advance for a "Team Deathmatch" game played at the Armageddon field. The design of the field was inspired by "Call of Duty", another one of my favorite video games; a simulation of infantry and World War II warfare. At Adrenaline Park, they created Armageddon field to look like a ravished warzone neighborhood with burnt cars, barrels and heavy duty truck tires scattered around. Deathmatch games consist of two teams. Of course, the objective of each team is to eliminate the players of the opponent one. I had tried several of the guns on my previous visits, and I enjoyed using the rifle gun. I planned to use it again today.

We arrived on time. In the parking lot of Adrenaline Park, Omar's cousin waited with the rest of the gang. A couple of years older than us, he drove his mother's car. When they saw us, the four guys stepped out of the car. With the exception of Omar's cousin, I knew the three other guys from school. Omar's cousin had already started college.

"You're the parkour guy?" Omar's cousin approached me

smiling.

I nodded and my eyes sparkled. I swelled with pride.

"I always wanted to play parkour."

I knew even if he did not want to play parkour, he had to say that. People like him, muscular and well-built took one shot at me and the first thing that pops in their minds is, if this fat boy can do it, I certainly can.

"You should give it a try," I said, "you will like it."

He asked me many questions about the game and its techniques. As I talked, everyone became interested to learn more about me and my training routines. They asked questions and listened attentively to me as I explained the game. I became the center of attention. I got the spotlight. I felt like the star of the show, and it felt awesome.

Their exhilaration intensified, and so did mine.

"Show us what you do," they asked.

"Show us some of your movements," they insisted.

Overwhelmed with excitement, I did not think twice to assess the situation. I ran forward at my normal speed to front flip. They all stood there watching me. To perform a front flip, one neither has to run fast or slow. Running fast throws you off balance and you fall. Running slow will not give you enough push to flip. I knew that by heart. I have trained relentlessly and I flipped hundreds of times before. I had mastered the move.

What I failed to assess though was that I ran on sandy ground, not the usual ground I trained on and became familiar with. On the sandy ground, my normal speed for flip needed adjustment, which within the feverish excitement, I overrode. As a result, I flipped in the air alright, but because I did not plant my feet on time before my jump; the jump was delayed. I flipped too soon. I twisted my leg in the air and I landed hard and wrong on my foot.

My right knee snapped, I had twisted it beyond its range of motion. I lost my balance and fell to the ground. Maybe it was the excitement, the adrenaline, my pumping heart or whatever, but I did not feel any pain. I stood up, dusted my clothes, feeling embarrassed. I could not understand how or why I did not land properly. I was not aware, yet, there is a different pace for each ground and that I had to adjust my pace accordingly.

I took a deep breath and I ran to dive roll, another move I had mastered. A dive roll movement is used to overcome obstacles. It is performed by jumping in the air, in a diving technique as if jumping into a swimming pool, but using the hand to control the landing. Then the player rolls on the ground and stands up.

I ran fast. My right knee was certainly injured, even though I did not feel the full impact of my injury yet. But by then the adrenaline started to fade, and as I prepared to jump, my right leg failed to push the ground. Instead of lunging forward, my body rolled and tilted, and as gravity pulled me, I fell on my right shoulder, with all my weight on top of it. I heard a loud crack, my shoulder.

I rolled on the ground, and in my shock, one last boost of adrenaline rushed through my body, enough to put me back on my feet. I stood up. My broken shoulder dangled in front of me, the bone protruded from the side of my arm. I started to cry in panic. All I could think of was my mother, and what she would do to me if she saw this. She didn't even know I was here. I feared her anger more than the pain I started to feel. I was scared. I cried, I wailed, I hyperventilated. My friends heard me cry, but they walked towards the entrance, leaving me behind, as if I did not exist. I cried louder and pleaded for someone to stay with me. Regretfully, they all declined. We had paid for the paintball park in advance, and no one wanted to miss the fun, or waste the money.

They disappeared inside the gate, and left me lying on the sidewalk with a broken shoulder and a torn meniscus. As my body cooled off, the pain intensified, both physically and emotionally. I sat there helpless, pitying myself and crying. An old man who worked there brought me a bag of ice. I put it on my knee. It did not help a bit. I called my dad. He arrived as fast as he could, two hours later, during which I waited alone on the sidewalk. None of my friends came out to check on me.

And by the time I left, they were still inside the park.

*

PART TWO
Silver Lining

THE TURNING POINT

"We generally change ourselves for one of two reasons: inspiration or desperation." —Jim Rohn

There are turning points in people's lives — either on the con-science or sub-conscience levels — after which people evolve and grow. There is always a Before *"this turning point"* and an After. No matter what its magnitude, effect or result is; if *"this turning point"* did not kill you, it certainly made you stronger. I am paraphrasing Friedrich Nietzsche's quote here. When you think about it, nothing really kills you, but death itself. Everything else transforms you.

The culmination of events, experiences and incidents that led to *"the turning point"* in your life, prepares you for what is coming ahead, moves your story forward, strengthens and impacts you, perhaps in a negative way, when you first look at it. In our desperation, we are short sighted to see that the negative impact is temporary. We become blinded by our own victimhood that we fail to grasp the changes happening in our lives. These changes bring life as we know it to an end. But that end should be celebrated not mourned, because it also marks a new beginning.

There is always a better life hovering around the corner ready to emerge, just waiting for a sign that we buried the old life. The one that had caused us nothing but agony and despair. Life waits for the choices we make. How we grow out of misery is our choice, and how we stay in it is also our choice. Some people prefer to bask in their feelings of sorrow and victimhood. They will stay there until they choose to change, on their own.

Of course, it was not easy to convince a 15-years-old staying in home confinement with his shoulder in a sling and his leg in a cast, that the accident — which he considered then the worst thing that had happened in his life — was actually the best thing. My 15-years-old self never saw it as a blessing, and not until years later when I contemplated life, its meaning and the events and incidents that shaped me. I must admit I sympathize with my younger self. The five months succeeding the accident were the culmination of every abuse, bullying, heartache, years of loneliness, despair and frustration. My younger self had had enough and chose to change.

After the accident, I was not only confined, but the knee and leg surgeries I underwent left me immobile and incapacitated. I had hit rock bottom with nowhere else to sink below that. Now, I know hitting rock bottom was the only way for me to bounce back. The harder one hits, the higher one bounces. Thus, my accident despite its outcome, was in fact a blessing in disguise, even though I did not know it then. Without the accident, I would never have had the motive, chance or will power to change. The fall that broke my shoulder, knee and foot was hard on me, both emotionally and physically. Yet, it was the sign for me to bury my old life. And because of the forcefulness of my fall, I bounced back high.

Motivational speaker, Jim Rohn, once said, "You cannot change the circumstances, the seasons or the wind, but you can change yourself. That is something you have charge of." I believe and agree with every word. Even though I did not know this quote then, I assert the accident became my turning point. The second turning point to be precise, for before it, came the basketball incident, but it was not as intense. Nonetheless, both incidents prepared me for the change. Sometimes we receive more than one sign, more than one chance.

I had my life before the accident, which I could not change, and my life after it, which was left up to me to shape. My incapacitation became my force for change. From the pain I suffered, both emotional and physical, and from the anguish, agony, despair and loneliness came the transformation. I was the caterpillar that turned into a butterfly. In the darkness of my isolation, my wings grew. Once the sling and cast were removed, I had transformed. I emerged as a butterfly ready for a new phase in my life.

*

I was in tenth grade when my friends abandoned me on the curb by the entrance of the paintball range. School had started a month earlier, and I had just turned 15. With a fractured shoulder, torn meniscus and a broken foot, I underwent few surgeries and spent five months at home to recover. I wore a shoulder sling for eight months, four of which my arm was tied to my body and tucked under my clothes.

After the surgery, I returned back from the hospital to my dark hole. I am not exaggerating when I say that during the five months of confinement, no one came to visit me. No one picked up the phone to call and see how I was doing, if I needed help with school work, or even if I were still alive. Not even the cool guys, the ones I considered them close to me. I had given them an excuse for leaving me on the curb and waking away. They had already paid for the paintball range and would have lost the money they had saved for the outing. I forgave them for leaving me behind that day, but I could not find an excuse for any of them not to call me after the surgery. They had five months to redeem themselves, but they did not, not even Karim. Well, I take it back. Karim called me twice or three times, not once he asked about my well-being, or if I needed anything. We mostly talked about video games.

If I had lied to myself up to this point, after my accident it became obvious that no one cared about me. To put it bluntly, not a single person gave a damn about me. I did not want anyone to pity me, I just wanted to feel I mattered in someone's life. Unfortunately, I did not. I was just a shadow in their lives. Someone they could easily dispose of like a paper tissue. And they did at the first opportunity. Even though it hurt so much, I must admit I did not expect a different behavior from them. They lived to my expectations. In a sense, they did not disappoint me, yet still deep in my heart, I wished, thought, hoped, someone would call me, pretend he cared.

Normally, I would have been able to walk with crutches after my knee surgery, but because of my shoulder injury, I could not put the top of the crutch under my right arm. These five months, I moved around by holding one crutch with my left hand and hopping around on one foot, mostly to the bathroom, as nowhere else was easily accessible to me. Every movement was hard; and with my limited mobility, showering, putting on clothes, standing up, sitting down were challenging, but nonetheless, I somehow managed on my own. And if you thought my pillow had seen enough tears before, you could not be more wrong.

Why, God, why? Why me? I asked these questions every day in my life ever since I could remember, ever since I became aware I was different. I never lived a normal childhood. I never had a friend. I endured humiliation by people I knew. Strangers in the streets bullied and harassed me. I became the butt of everyone's joke. I lived in isolation my entire life. I felt like an outsider, an outcast, with no one to turn to for help or support. No one could feel my pain. Everyone avoided me as if I had contracted a contagious disease. At 15, when life finally started smiling at me, when I made friends who accepted me, included me in their plans and invited me to their outings, life punched me in the face once again, even harder than before.

Until then, my life had been nothing but a series of heartaches, sufferings and many unanswered questions. I lived in a prison made of flesh and blood, and a lot of fat; My body had become my prison. I asked God for explanations, but He never gave me any. I prayed every night, asked Him to help me lose weight, stop eating, let people be kind to me. I asked Him what I did to suffer that much, but He never answered my prayers or my questions. He never gave me explanations at that time because He had bigger plans for me later.

I could not comprehend why life treated me unfairly. I questioned why circumstances were against me, why I did not have friends and why the friends I thought I had abandoned me and walked away when I needed them the most. In the confinement of my home, and as I marinated in victimhood, my anger and frustration escalated with every passing day. I was angry at myself, at people, at life, at the orthopedic surgeon who told me I would never be able to run or play sports again. I was angry at the physiotherapist who blamed me for my injuries, because "FAT boys should not play these sports." I was angry at my mother, and all along, I never stopped wondering why God chose me to be fat.

After I hit rock bottom – feeling crushed, my life destroyed and with nothing in the forecast but pain, loneliness and isolation – all I could think of was I wanted to recover and go back to play parkour. I did not know how I was going to play parkour when I could not even move my arm an inch, but in my desperate condition, that was all I could think of. For a right handed, this made studying even harder. During this time, I taught myself to write with my left hand, and that is how I did my homework. It was hard and I struggled with it, like I struggled with everything else, but I liked the fact that I learned to write with my left hand. It made me realize that I can learn anything I want if I put my mind into it. I vowed to change. I vowed to lose weight. I did not know how, but I wanted to recover and lose weight to be able to play parkour again. Parkour became an obsession, my number one motivation for weight loss. But there was also another more important reason, a personal one. I wanted people to appreciate me and to love me. In my mind, I knew they would only do that if I lost weight.

Over the years, with my meager knowledge about health and nutrition, I perpetually tried to lose weight on my own. I dieted many times and failed, because I could not commit to any diet long enough to see results. After the accident, I became determined to lose weight. I just did not know how to start or what I should do. Every day I woke up with good intentions. Every day I started a new diet, decreased my food intake, and tried to keep my mouth closed. I succeeded for most of the day, but eventually I would lose control, binge or go on an eating spree. I would start again the following day, and it went on and on and on, like Groundhog Day.

For emotional eaters, diets do not really work all the time, and committing to a diet is the hardest thing to do. Emotional eaters, which I am one of them, we do not eat when we are hungry and we do not stop eating because we are full. Food helps us cope with our sorrows and anxieties. It comforts and soothes us. Once we start eating, food triggers our addiction and we cannot stop. This is why diets do not work on the long term, but changing eating habits do. But at 15, I did not know any of that. Thus, despite how much I tried to diet in the five months of home confinement, I miserably failed every time and naturally, I lost zero grams. Yet, I did not get discouraged as I always did because I was adamant to lose weight at any cost.

As it turned out, success is the culmination of failures, and I had failed a lot. But this time I had set my mind, either succeed or die. I had no other choice. I did not want to live the rest of my life trapped in this body. I became adamant to escape from it, lose it somewhere where it would never find me back. I did not want to spend the rest of my life with the label "fat" stuck on me.

Thus, the choice was clear: diet or die.

After five months of forced rest, the orthopedic removed the leg cast and gave me permission to go back to school. My shoulder was still in a sling, but untied from my body. With the clearance to leave the house, I also started physiotherapy. I went to the physiotherapist three times a week where I spent two long painful hours each visit; one hour for my shoulder and one for my leg. The physiotherapist told me I would never play parkour again. He blamed me for my injuries, because "FAT boys should not play these sports." Announcing the end of my parkour-mania crushed me. It shattered my life to pieces. Labeling me fat angered me. His words still ring in my ears until today. One would expect demeaning labels and judgmental statements from bullies at school, but not from his physiotherapist. Nonetheless, I did not allow his words to discourage me. I had already activated the *succeed or die mode*, and had embarked on my journey to change.

*

LIFE CHANGING DECISION

Waiting for my turn at the nutrition clinic filled me with apprehension. Visiting a dietitian was the last thing I expected myself to do, yet my last resort after all attempts to lose weight on my own failed. I had mixed feelings though. On the one hand, I desperately looked forward and anticipated a positive outcome, even though I did not know how the dietitian would succeed to stop me from eating. On the other hand, the idea of meeting with him filled me with fear and anxiety. I did not want to see more eyes humiliating me, making fun of my weight. I did not want to hear more lectures, or worse, I did not want him to deprive me from my favorite food. Food has been my companion throughout my life. Just the thought of taking it away overwhelmed me with separation anxiety. How could I give away my best friend? We had been inseparable until then.

Despite my apprehension, I enjoyed the soft music playing in the background. More overweight and obese clients sat around the waiting area, comparing diets and laughing together. No one seemed to notice me or my classmate Walid, who sat next to me, waiting for his turn too. Overweight himself, he came up with the idea to consult a dietitian. At school, we had talked together about our weight problems, shared notes about our difficulties and challenges to lose it.

I wiped my sweaty palms with a tissue and clasped them together to stop my hands from shaking. I took a deep breath to slow down my racing heart and focused my gaze at a pin up calendar with a photo of green mountains, somewhere, with the name of a pharmaceutical company printed on it.

The ceiling fan whirled over my head. Three other young adults waited with their parents. Two boys my age waited with their mothers. A younger obese girl sat next to her overweight father. Both had red hair and freckles. She flipped through the pages of a glossy celebrities' magazine. Above her hung a poster with bright colorful fruits and vegetables; broccoli, carrots, apples, bananas and other of my least favorite foods. My crystal ball told me these food items would be my destiny for a while.

Walid and I were the only ones unaccompanied by adults. Technically we were under age, not that anyone enforced it, but we had come with the recommendations of his mother, also one of the dietitian's clients. In fact, she had been nagging Walid for a while to visit the dietitian. When he suggested to me to go along, I welcomed the idea, an option I had never considered before, out of ignorance mostly. When he presented it to me, I got excited and even wondered why I never thought about it before. After hitting rock bottom, I had nothing to lose. I found no harm to try. On the contrary, I was curious about this new experience. The dietitian may know something I did not, obviously. If I succeeded, it would be a great achievement for me. If I did not, I would be back where I started. A place I was not comfortable in, but familiar with.

Walid's mother called the dietitian's office and made the appointments for us, to make sure he went. From my end, I hid my plan from my mother. She did not think highly of dietitians and firmly believed that until the age of 21, a diet might stop my growth. Unfortunately, that is the culture I grew up in. Her answer to my dilemma was to close my mouth and eat reasonably, to take responsibility for my own weight and not to seek help from others. Why could not I just do it myself, she asked.
As if I had not tried tens of times before.

My relationship with my mother was complicated to start with, and after the accident, it worsened. With both my siblings married, and my father's long working hours and traveling, she had no one to dump her anger and frustration on, but me. While confined at home for five months, I lived in guilt and shame. Every day she blamed me for what happened. She did not miss a chance to remind me that I brought it upon myself, it was all my fault. Not to mention the continuous scolding for going behind her back. Her company became intolerable, yet no one else took care of me but her. She helped me physically, but mentally and emotionally she tormented me.

To avoid her, I hardly left my room. I even stopped joining my parents at the dinner table when my father was around. Since we had a distant relationship to start with, neither of us minded not spending dinner time together. The dinner table had become a family battle ground, anyway. My mother divided her blame between my father and I, but her arguments with my father usually escalated and turned ugly. Dinner time with them became a stressful and unpleasant experience. I enjoyed my own company more than spending time in theirs.

The girl with freckles sitting across the waiting area at the dietitian's office looked up from the glossy magazine. She caught me looking in her direction. In my deep thoughts, I probably looked like I gazed at her. We made eye contact and she smiled at me. I froze for an awkward moment. I rubbed my sweaty palms and before I knew what to do, she turned her head away, and tucked it back into the magazine. I knew I should have smiled back at her, but I was too embarrassed.

I went to a mixed school, but I never had the courage to talk to a girl, not even my classmates, let alone smile at one. Ashamed and embarrassed of myself and how I looked in their eyes, I feared their rejection. I never put myself in any situation where a girl would reject even smiling back at me. I kept a low profile and avoided any encounter with them.

*

THE WORST THING IN LIFE CAN BECOME THE BEST THING IN LIFE

After two visits to the dietitian, Walid lost interest and disappeared, but I continued my journey which I started at 15 with a weight of 135 kg. I met the dietitian once a week, on Mondays. He measured my waist, weighed me and wrote me a new diet. Despite the strict diet he put me on, he advised me against playing sports. He told me that exercise while in the process of losing weight will grow my muscles, which in turn will slow down the weight loss. This is completely false, but back then I did not know any better. Nonetheless, I used my common sense and I exercised anyway.

It took me a month of strict diet to see results. At the beginning, I convinced my mother that I was dieting on my own, but later I told her the truth. She scolded me as usual, but then accepted the fact when she saw my determination. Meanwhile, two things happened to me. Firstly, I stumbled into the Insanity Program, a complete guide to nutrition and workout, mostly cardio, offered by personal trainer Shaun T and his team. You follow the workout videos from anywhere, and I did. It was my first time to try these exercises and I greatly enjoyed them. Not to mention they helped me drop a lot of weight.

In addition, during this time I also became interested to learn more about nutrition. The dietitian's knowledge intrigued me. He knew everything about nutrition and dieting from the top of his head, and he wrote me the food plan without checking any references or guidebooks. His knowledge and information about food and calories fascinated me. He knew precisely what I should eat and the adequate amounts I needed to drop the weight I desired. In my mind, he was either a con artist setting me up to financially take advantage of me, or a magician. But he was neither, just an expert in his field. I became curious to learn how he knew what works for me. Why he suggests I eat this and not that. I wanted to know how he calculated the quantities I had to consume, to lose a certain amount of weight. I wanted to know why I need protein and not carbs, why I avoid sugar and substitute fat, and why eating McDonalds made me gain weight while salads did not. I was clueless and keen to learn the science behind nutrition and to understand how to implement it on me. He knew what worked for me, and I also wanted to learn what worked for me.

I exhausted Google and YouTube for answers to my inquiries. Between both, I found abundant information about health, nutrition and exercise. I lost 30 kg in six months. In the first four months, I lost 20 kg with the help of the dietitian. By then, I had acquired a lot of knowledge and wanted to experiment on my own. I stopped going to the dietitian and lost 15 more kg, by following the routine I developed.

When I started college at 18, I weighed 85 kg, three kilos away from my target weight. By the time I reached my target weight, I had lost a total of 53 kg.

*

Everyone complimented me on the miracle I accomplished. Elated by this achievement myself, I had to explain to them that miracles do not just happen. Goals are achieved by hard work and perseverance. Big successes are the result of even bigger failures and sacrifices. And more important than the weight I lost on this journey of transformation was what I had gained. I gained insight, knowledge, determination and a purpose for life.

I meet many people who are suffering from the same dilemma. To them I say, "You are not alone. I hear you. I feel for you. I understand what you have been through. I have been there myself. You are not alone anymore. I am here to offer you moral support and share with you my experience."

Before I went to the dietitian my life consisted of a series of failures. Topping the list was my continuous struggle with weight and the failure to lose it. Naturally, the obvious cause for my obesity was I consumed large quantities of food. I also binged between meals. I did not go out of my way to binge, but if food was served or put in front of me at irregular hours, for any reason, I did not turn it down. The vast majority of people eat between meals. Eating between meals is not an exclusive trait of overweight people, but binging is. The meaning of binging is to eat excessively over a period of time, lose control over the food and then feel guilty after it. And, while not all people who binge are obese, unfortunately, all obese people binge. The difference between people with normal weight and obese people, judging from my own experience, is the amount of food each group consumes and the binging frequency. Friends may meet at a party on a weekend, eat and drink excessively for a few hours and then go home. This is not binging. In my case, I did enough damage at meal times that binging between meals was certainly a factor that contributed to my problem, but not the direct cause of it.

Gaining and losing weight follows a simple mathematical equation. It is all about calories intake vs calories burned. If you eat more calories than you burn, you gain weight. If you eat less calories than you burn, you lose weight. If your calories intake equals the calories you burn, you neither lose nor gain weight. Of course, there are other factors that contribute to the storage of fat in our bodies, like age and metabolism. But for young obese people who wonder why they gained so much weight, I hate to repeat bluntly to them what they already know, but hope to hear another reason; "You are obese because you eat more than you burn. Period."

*

FOOD ADDICTION

Before I embarked on the nutrition awakening journey, my meals consisted of heaps and heaps of high calorie foods, and I could not control the portions. I ate everything served in front of me. Overeaters and food addicts have different eating patterns and behaviors around food than normal eaters and non-addicts. Overeaters and food addicts neither eat because they are hungry nor stop eating when they are full. Their perception of hunger is distorted from that of normal people.

People who have no eating disorders do not eat unless they are hungry and they stop eating when they are full. On the other hand, food addicts eat because there is food in front of them. They stop eating when food is taken away from them, realistically devoured by them, because compulsive overeaters and food addicts will not allow anyone to take away their food. Just look at a swarm of locusts attacking and devouring the crops. Watch the damage they create as they leave nothing behind. Now imagine the eating behavior of food addicts and compulsive overeaters when they are surrounded by food. They would attack open buffets just like locusts attack the crops. In restaurants, they leave no leftovers. You will never see them walk out of restaurants with doggie bags. They may even eat the food left by their company. Leftovers do not go to waste. Not on their watch. I know exactly how they behave, for that is also how I behaved around food.

Growing up, I ate larger portions of food than what a child my age needed for growth or physical activity. I also lived a sedentary life. The result was disastrous. At the age of 15, I carried the weight of two people my age, combined. Naturally, my diet consisted of high calorie unhealthy and junk food. All food is healthy when consumed at the right amount. Our bodies need carbs, protein and even fat. But what most people do not understand is that whatever calories our bodies do not burn, they are converted into fat and stored as such. As a child, I could devour a whole oven pan of baked pasta with gooey sauces and melted cheeses. I licked clean the pots and pans. Comfort food always soothes me and there is a reason why it is called as such.

While I am powerless over food in general, I am addicted to cheeses. Pasta with cheese, pizza with extra cheese, cheese sandwiches, plain cheese. I added mountains of cheese on whatever I ate, and I would not stop eating until the mountain was leveled to the ground. Ironically, and unlike most obese people, deserts did not contribute much to my obesity. For some odd reason, I do not have a sweet tooth. Nonetheless, I did enough damage to myself and my health without it. But with the exception of deserts, which I ate at lesser amounts, my diet included every other food item and I consumed food inhumanly.

My eating behavior and patterns are not out of the ordinary for addicts. Food is an addictive substance just like drugs or alcohol. Addicts of various substances consume their substance of addiction without thinking, food addicts included. They follow the same pattern. They eat first and then think of the damage they inflicted on themselves when it is already too late. While addicts of other substances are invisible to the masses, the extra weight obese people carry around gives them away. People cross path with drug addicts, gamblers and alcoholics without noticing them, but they will notice the shadow of an obese person a mile away. If an obese person steps in the elevator with them, they will start wondering if the elevator load exceeded its limit. They will hold their breath until the elevator safely reaches its destination. An obese person knows exactly what goes through the minds of people when they see him. People should learn to be kind to obese people for they are struggling to fit in the world. They are not happy with the excess weight they carry even though they pretend to be impartial about it or pretend they do not care. And please spare them the rhetorical question of why do not they go on a diet. Do you think they are not trying to diet every single day of their lives?

Food addiction is an eating disorder. It is important

to mention that not all people with eating disorders are overweight or obese. Some bulimics may be food addicts who maintain their weight by purging or non-purging methods. Food addicts could also be people who exercise excessively, who burn more calories than they consume and that is how they maintain their weight, despite the fact that they experience the emotional symptoms and suffer from the side effects that accompany their addiction. Food addicts come in various shapes and forms, and emotional baggage.

It is equally important to mention that not all overweight people are food addicts. Weight creeps on for various reasons, especially as people get older and their physical activities and metabolism slow down. Normal people, who do not suffer from eating disorders, and who were not obese children or adults, might find themselves gaining weight as they age. They might gain a lot of weight over a decade. They take action to drop it. They reduce their calorie intake, go to a nutritionist or dietitian for a few weeks or months to speed up the process, or add exercise to their daily routine. They eventually lose the extra weight and move on with their lives. They might repeat that every few years to maintain their weight, for body image or to avoid health issues.

*

The difference between normal people who gain weight and food addicts is simple to explain. For normal people, food is the fuel they need to carry on with their daily life activities. They use food for energy. The function of food to them stops there. They eat, get the energy they need, use it until they run out of energy, and then replenish it by eating another meal with sufficient calories to sustain their lives and activities. Normal people are like cars. Cars do not store fuel. You take your car to the gas station when the tank is empty. For normal people, the kitchen is the gas station. They eat only when they are hungry, when their tank is empty. They will stop eating when they are full. That was another eye-opening revelation I learned on my weight loss journey.

I lived my entire life up to the first visit to the dietitian as a monster, or as many labeled me; a freak. With his help, I chained the beast inside me and transformed myself into a car, and used fuel as needed. I went through a hard and challenging transition. From my previous failures to lose weight, I knew I lacked the determination to adhere to an eating plan long enough to achieve results. But this time I had enough determination to go through it. Everyone who knew me, knew of my ill determination in general, and specifically of my weakness towards food. I grew tired of how they viewed and labeled me.

I wanted to prove them all wrong. Proving them wrong was what motivated me to lose weight, and propelled me to stay the course until I succeeded. I wanted to show them I was not the loser they thought of, and that I had the willpower and determination to change the course of my life and make a difference after all. Even though it was wrong to need to change for others, at that time I did not care. This need to change motivated me enough to take action, and that was what mattered. The end justifies the means.

I also wanted to change because I grew tired of who I became. I often wonder if I hadn't been bullied, labeled or shamed, would I have gone through the trouble to change my body and thus my image? Probably not. But we are living in a society that judges people by their looks. I understand living a healthy life in a healthy body is important on more than one level. I never regretted the transition in my life, but under different circumstances, I would have been content with who I was — not who I became. Not everyone wants to be athletic, with wide shoulders and a six pack. Many young people, both males and females are driven to look their best because of how their image is perceived by others — not because it is what they want. Do not get me wrong. If this perfect body image is what they strive for, and to achieve it they spend a large part of their lives exercising, more power to them and I wish them all the best. I am merely expressing my dismay at the social stereotypes that drive young people to live by the expectations of others, not their own. I want people of all ages to be content with their body image, comfortable in their own skin, literally — to accept who they are, how they look, and to feel good about themselves, no matter what their weight is. This is our responsibility as human beings towards each other, to break these molds and lift each other up.

With the help of my dietitian, my determination and motivation to adhere to a food plan lasted longer than the previous times. What differed this time was I had him to guide me and I reported to him my progress each week. If you have tried to lose weight on your own several times and failed, there is nothing wrong to seek professional help. Because I had to report to the dietitian my weekly success or failure, that in itself helped me adhere to the food plan he prescribed to me. If I messed it up, he scolded me. He held me accountable for every bite I ate. This helped me later to develop a strategy and I continued to follow it on my own after I stopped seeing him.

*

WHY DID THE DIET WORK?

In the duration of the two months I spent with the dietitian, I abided by the food plan he prescribed for me. For six consecutive days, I measured and weighed my food, counted the calories and ate the exact portions. The seventh day was a free day. I ate what my heart desired. The plan was not the ideal, but somehow, as most chemical diets, it curbed my cravings and controlled my hunger, to a substantial degree. The combinations of food reacted together and hence cravings became less intense. It could all be mental too. Who knows? After repeating something for too long, it becomes a habit.

    I bought a little booklet where I kept a food journal. I also wrote down everything I craved during the restricted six days of dieting. On my free day, I ate the list of food I wrote in my journal during the week. This helped my abstinence — The fact that I was not deprived from this food item for the rest of my life made me tolerate my short-term craving. I saw the light at the end of each week. Eating these items was also my reward. On my free day, I celebrated my little achievement with my friends. We went out to eat, of course. It became our ritual. Because it is hard to uninstall old habits and re-install new ones, it was both difficult and challenging for me at the beginning to stick to a diet. To help me install these new habits, I put a condition for myself. If I did not maintain my discipline and abstinence for six days, I deprived myself from the reward on my free day. I had to wait for the following week to satisfy my cravings.

On my weight loss journey, I discovered the power of the human brain and how it works in mysterious ways. In addition, I also discovered we have power over our brain — whatever we install becomes who we are. Some say it takes three weeks to install a new habit, some say three months. From my experience, it took me something in between a month and a half and two months to rewire my brain and recondition myself to stick to my new eating habits, that I had practiced up to that point. It was not easy to stop eating the food I loved, limit the portion, or resist the temptation of eating a freshly baked cake coming out of the oven. It was pure torture to walk by a fast food place and resist the temptation of walking in, no matter how much the wafting aromas tickled my senses. None of that was easy. Declining a desert after dinner or a slice of cake with coffee is not a behavior food addicts and compulsive overeaters would normally do. Thus, each accomplishment was a milestone that required celebration and a pat on the shoulder.

While losing weight is hard, on the other hand, gaining it is easy as pie, and as delicious as one too. It is easy to gain weight because we have acquired many bad eating habits that we continue to do unconsciously. For example, eating large buckets of popcorn with butter at the movies is a habit we acquired and continue to do so because everyone else does it. By identifying these bad habits, we can un-learn-them the same way we learned them.

My visits to the dietitian opened my eyes at so many levels. I benefited from these visits more than just losing the weight. I did not learn anything specific about nutrition, though, but the doctor inspired me by what he did. The way he grouped the food for me, in a way that made me lose weight, fascinated me. He wrote food plans that I followed and I shed weight in the process. I had no discipline when it came to food and for the first time in my life, I realized that discipline was all I needed. He introduced me to abstinence; the act of refraining from compulsive eating, and showed me how a food plan can help me achieve my abstinence. In brief, he helped me install the new habit of eating normal amounts of food, both in quality and quantity.

His knowledge intrigued me to learn more about this science, and about food and my body. I wanted to learn for myself, to be able to understand my weight problem, to be able to solve or cope with it. I did not imagine myself going to dietitians for the rest of my life, but at the same time I was also fully aware of my weakness and powerlessness over food. I had enough sense to realize that no matter how much weight I lose, if I was left to my own vices, without being careful, or working hard to maintain the weight loss, I will gain it back. Thus, I developed a backup plan, acquired the knowledge I would need when I am on my own.

My curiosity led me back to google, my best and trusted friend. There, I found abundant information about food and nutrition that satisfied my curiosity. This information also led me to YouTube, my other friend. Hungry for knowledge, no pun intended, beyond what was available on online, I signed up for online courses. I bought the textbooks, studied hard and became a certified personal trainer at the age of 17, probably the youngest in Egypt then. This certification was a milestone in my life, in the career I did not know yet I would be starting. It is interesting how life shapes us before we even realize it. When I look back at all the misfortunes in my life, I realize they happened for a purpose and I was brought to life for a mission bigger than myself. The pain, humiliation, and suffering I had gone through were to prepare me for what was coming ahead.

*

Compulsive overeating is a disease - an incurable one. In other words, no one is cured from compulsive overeating and food addiction. People who are born in the clutches of the disease are destined to live with it for the rest of their lives. More bad news; As I mentioned earlier, food addiction is the hardest. It is harder than drug, alcohol or gambling addiction. The reason for that is because other addicts can stop or distance themselves from the substance they abuse and live an addiction free life. Food addicts on the other hand need food to survive, despite food is the substance they abuse and the cause of their problems. In other words, while food addicts are advised to stop eating compulsively, they still have to eat to live.

This makes abstinence hard for many. How can you abstain from a substance that you need to survive? As a result, food addicts slip more than people with other addictions. It is hard to stop thinking of food when you are tasting its flavors or when its wafting aromas trigger your desire to eat.

Eat - do not eat - you can eat this, but you cannot eat that. This ambiguity leads to a lot of confusion. Confusion leads to stress and anxiety, and both lead to eating, and overeating. Until today, I am still powerless over food. I constantly think of it. Some days more than others, but as other food addicts, I am generally obsessed with food than not. My relationship with food has been the longest and the most sustainable in my life. It took different shapes and forms over the years. It changed, mutated, transformed, but nonetheless, it is the constant factor in my life.

Growing up, my life rotated around food. Food is my escapism. It is everything beautiful in life. It soothes me, helps me forget my troubles, eases my pain. Food makes my life happier. It makes me a happier person. It is my life long buddy, my best friend, and my faithful and loyal companion. When everyone else abandons me, food is there for me. Eating helps me cope with whatever problems or hardships life throws at me. Socially. Professionally. Emotionally. Financially. You name it. For many years, food controlled me and I wholeheartedly surrendered to it. I must admit it is still controlling me to a certain extent, but now I have the tools and knowledge that help me resist and cope with it. I win sometimes, I lose at other times, and the struggle continues. But I do not allow food to control me for longer than it should.

*

There is no problem or trouble, a double order of Big Mac with extra fries drowning in ketchup and washed down with chocolate shake, cannot make you forget. But looking at the big picture objectively, food never solved any of my problems. It only suppressed the anxiety caused by this problem. Drug addicts use drugs to alter their reality. Food alters my reality too. The sad thing is that after I overeat, the problem that triggered my food compulsion and overeating in the first place does not disappear. It is still there looming over my head, waiting for an action to be taken. Food just soothed my injured ego and calmed my anxiety, temporarily, but fixed nothing. Moreover, I feel guilty for eating over it.

This guilt can put me down on my knees and cry; regretting what I did, fretting on my powerlessness over food. Food addiction is a cunning and baffling disease. It attacks when people are at their weakest points, when their guards are down. The good news is, the more I learned about myself, my body, my eating habits and patterns, I became able to identify the signs and symptoms of the disease. This taught me to resist and fight back. Yes, it is an ongoing struggle, a non-ending battle, unfortunately.

Compulsive eating often disguises in the form of hunger pangs. If I am keeping my abstinence and following my food plan, eating at the assigned times the quantity I measured and weighed, I know there is no reason for me to be hungry. This way, hunger does not deceive me, and I do not feed it. Often we feel hungry when we are not. Hunger pang is a spike, a brain signal. So is thirst. On many occasions, the body even confuses thirst for hunger. Sometimes the answer to hunger pangs is just drinking a glass of water to quench the thirst, or just ignore it.

*

MENTAL GAMES

The brain of a food addict plays a lot of tricks for the person to eat. And being an addict myself, food thoughts never elude me. Every single day of my life, I am bombarded with thoughts to overeat, eat the wrong things, or eat at times when I am not supposed to eat, like when I am full for example. There is no one way to live with food addiction or compulsive eating. Also, there is no right or wrong way to try to lose weight and maintain it. Each person knows what is best for him. What works for one may not necessarily work for the other. For weight loss, like everything else in life, there is no absolute. From my own experience, I admit that food journaling and planning my meals helped me stick to my plan.

Obviously, and it goes without saying, I slipped a lot over the years and I still do. It is normal. We are only humans. And that is what humans do. They fall, get up, keep going and keep trying. Slipping means breaking the abstinence, binging between meals, eating items not on my food plan, overeating, or all of the above. Slipping is a reminder that my disease is incurable. At the beginning when I slipped, I used to beat myself hard. I would go on guilt trips that decanted and almost destroyed me. Then, I learned guilt is a toxic feeling. It does not resolve the problem, but rather intensifies it.

When something or someone triggers in me negative emotions, my first defense mechanism to deal with the pain these feelings arouse in me is to eat, and overeat. As I mentioned a while ago, food is soothing. Food is the anesthesia of the soul. It temporarily numbs the pain, but of course it does not heal the wound. Food numbs my injured soul, puts to sleep the negative emotions; hurt, fear, anger, anxiety, humiliation and whatever degrading feelings overwhelm me.

My immediate reaction when a negative feeling overwhelmed me was to eat over it. By the time I finished binging, and once the anesthesia that numbed the soul wore off, I was confronted with the reality that the problem that caused this episode is still persisting. Well of course, other than trying to pamper my injured soul with food, I had taken no action to face or resolve the issue that triggered these feelings in the first place. But now, in addition to feeling hurt, I am also swarmed with guilt feelings for overeating.

Binging at the time of anger is done subconsciously, senselessly. In this state of mind, as the hand goes from food to mouth, one does not stop to think, "What am I doing?" until a large bag of cookies, potato chips or a casserole of comfort food disappears. Before the brain stops you, damage is already done.

The guilt feelings that proceed these actions lead to despair, which lead to victimization, and it goes without saying, the result is more eating.

It took me years to learn to identify these symptoms. When I am hit by a sudden urge to eat, at a time I am not hungry or out of the routine, I stop and assess the reason that triggered this urge. First question I ask myself is, "Am I really hungry?" If it is not a meal time and I have followed my eating plan, I know I am not. So instead of eating, I take a moment to replay the thoughts and events that triggered the urge to eat. Do not be surprised when I tell you anything can trigger this urge for food addicts.

Perhaps a dispute with the boss over work performance, an argument with a friend, a loved one or one's mother. Watching one's football team loses a game. At other times, a casual or random thought might trigger it, like remembering an unresolved argument with your sibling that had happened years ago, or how a waiter answered back to you when your dessert was late, or a bullying incident at school when you were six years old. You will be amazed at what our minds can remind us of.

Often the reasons for our anxieties are legitimate. Feeling insecure about a job or a break up with the significant other are serious issues, but that does not justify overeating over them. Most people we meet in our life are going through serious hardships, but they do not eat. This is the difference between a normal person and one with eating disorders. For us food addicts, past incidents that once caused us anxiety, and unsolved issues pushed to the back of our minds, revisit us every once in a while. Our brains use them to trigger our disease.

Food addicts and people with other addictions or compulsive behaviors are walking on eggshells, for anything can cause them to slip. This is why it is important to realize what is going on and to be aware and cautious at all times of the tricks our brains play on us. And instead of dwelling on the problem, take action to resolve it. Whatever pain it takes to resolve a problem, in the long run it is less painful than falling in the clutches of the disease of addiction. Once addiction swallows us, it becomes harder to swim back to the shore safely. The longer we stay in this phase, the more we sink deeper into despair and helplessness, the feelings the disease thrives on.

*

THE VICTIMHOOD SYNDROME

Victimhood is an evident result of the disease of food addiction. Over the years and before I became aware of my addiction, I believed overeating was my problem. I could not have been more wrong. Overeating resulted from my problem. I gained weight because I overate. I overate because I had emotional problems that required attention, which I ignored. As I overate and gained weight, I looked at my life from my own prism. I believed the problems in my life were a result of being overweight. I hated myself and how I looked. The more I hated myself, the more I ate and gained weight. I blamed everyone else for my problems. I blamed my parents for passing over to me bad genes, my siblings for not understanding me enough, my teachers for letting the other kids bully me. I blamed life for being unfair. I prayed to God every night to enable me to eat like everyone else without gaining weight. When my prayers were not answered, I was angry.

I had reached a pathetic state where I even blamed my friends for eating in front of me. I was naive and delusional not to realize that my eating habits caused my weight gain, or that normal people with normal weight do not eat the amounts of food I consumed. In my sick mind, I believed the cosmic power conspired against me and prevented me from losing weight, even though I exercised vigorously. I also believed this same power messed up my diet, and forced me to eventually give it up. I became too absorbed in my own sorrows and victimhood to realize it was my fault, and mine alone. I was blind to see I had to change, make a difference. The more I learned, I stopped blaming life for my failures. Life gave everybody the same chance. I chose to overeat. My friends had all the right to eat whatever and whenever they wanted. I learned I cannot and should not control what people want to do or eat. If my friends hadn't tempted me, others would have. I cannot stop people from going on with their lives just because watching them eat offended me, or because they do not follow what I believe is good for me.

And naturally the cosmic power did not prevent me from losing weight despite my vigorous exercise, my eating habits did — once I learned about the calories equation, I acquitted the cosmic power. It goes without saying, no matter how vigorously I exercised, my calories intake exceeded the energy I burnt, and only when I reduced the calories I saw results.

The biggest challenge I faced on my weight loss journey

was to rewire my brain, uninstall the false beliefs and install new ones. In succeeding to do so, I found my purpose in life. I wanted to tell my story to the world. I wanted to transform people's lives the same way I transformed mine. Discovering this purpose motivated me to stop eating. By inspiring and motivating others, I also inspired and motivated myself.

At the age of 17, I had already been on my transformational journey for almost two years. I had achieved outstanding results and my business, SWAT, was flourishing. To the best of my knowledge, I was the youngest entrepreneur in the field of sports in Egypt.

When I started college, SWAT had already been in operation for three months.

*

EGYCON – MY FAIRYTALE

The cab stopped on the main road leading to the Greek Campus. We scooted out and walked around the corner to the gate, following the footsteps of the super heroes ahead of us on the shady sidewalk. The crisp morning sent chills down my spine. Jasmine walked next to me with fast strides. She pulled her gray raincoat tightly around her body, as if to trap the warmth of the sun that had radiated through the cab window on our way. She looked like a detective from an old TV show. I wanted to walk faster to a sunny spot, but even with her faster pace, I had to slow down to keep up with her.

Mortal Kombat's Sub-Zero and Scorpion hurried by, engaged in deep conversation, like best friends, oblivious of the staring eyes of people who stopped on the other side of the street to watch. Or maybe they consciously ignored them. A sober moment to see neither of them trying to stab or kill the other, as they would normally do in video games.

Cars driving by slowed down to watch the eccentric pedestrians dressed up in unusual costumes. No, Halloween didn't come in February. They were just cosplayers attending EGYcon.

Children inside the cars watched in disbelief. Their eyes popping at the sight of the super heroes. SpongeBob, walking ahead of us, waved at them. SpongeBob! What's he doing here? The children squealed in excitement and waved back at him. I guess he's somebody's hero too. The children bounced in their seats, their faces glued to the rear window as the cars drove away.

With my soaring excitement to reach my destination, I speeded up. Jasmine trotting behind me with larger strides. I've been waiting in anticipation to meet my super heroes too, and finally EGYcon made it happen. However, I was not just excited to meet them, I was one myself.

Pedestrians stood on the other side of the road watching and wondering what's going on, a rare sight to see grownups dressed in costumes and walking downtown Cairo. A couple of young men couldn't contain their curiosity and crossed over. Behind my shoulder I saw them talking with Kakashi, from the Japanese Naruto series, with his silver white spiky wig, leaf village headband and mask.

Attending EGYcon 2016 was a dream come true to many, including myself. I had already started the second semester of my first year in college, when I saw its poster on the billboard of one of the clubs I joined. Egypt's third annual anime, game and comic con was my first to attend. A full day event organized at the AUC Greek Campus, downtown on the first Saturday of February. Excited to attend, I bought my ticket weeks in advance. I would have never missed this event. I even created my own costume.

Around the corner, a vibrant crowd gathered in a sunny spot by the entrance of the Greek Campus. Music came from inside the walls of the campus and energized the crowd. The sun finally thawed me while we waited for our turn to walk in. I savored its warmth. Jasmine let go of her coat and rubbed her hands together to warm them, smiling at me with her bright green eyes; almost the same color of the eyes of the kitten I adopted two weeks earlier. Jasmine wore the colored lenses and red wig for the occasion. I could not understand the significance of the green eyes, red wig and the grey overcoat, but did not think it was appropriate to ask, so I left it there.

Stepping inside the gate of the Greek Campus teleported me to a scene in a video game, where the super heroes came to life. Actually, it looked like several video games and movies got tangled together and their characters were on break time. Not only that, but foes and adversaries walked together like best friends, and most probably they were.

The crowd exceeded my expectations. Knowing the capacity of the campus, there were at least 3000 people attending. Walking among superheroes, action figures, video gamers, otakus, cosplayers, anime and comic lovers was a dream come true.

Hitman with his red tie walked by, waving his two guns in the air. He passed us, and sure enough, he had the barcode tattoo printed on the back of his head. He stopped to talk to a reporter who walked around with a video camera and interviewed the characters.

The dark mesh blindfold slightly decreased my peripheral vision, and with the crowds around I bumped into people as we walked, but eventually found my rhythm. But Jasmine, who treated me like I was visually impaired, grabbed my hand and led me to the main stage where her friend Emma performed. On the way, we passed several Ninjas, a couple of Batmen, Kylo Ren from Star Wars, a few robots, and many characters I never saw before. They wore their appropriate costumes, capes, leather and body armors, and carried shiny swords, daggers, plastic machine guns from toy stores, scepters and foam weapons wrapped in aluminum foil and shimmered in the sun. It was fascinating to watch Japanese action figures mingling with Marvel characters. Two different cultures taking by storm young people of a third, an optimal definition of globalization. A comics and Marvel Universe fan, and a video gamer myself, I felt like a child in a candy store.

My heart skipped a beat when I saw Ezio from Assassin's Creed, with his white robe, hoodie and wrist knives, posing to the camera of a magazine that came to cover the event. I remembered all the good times we spent together and the pain I felt when I had to part with his video games. I hoped his new friend enjoyed him as much as I did. I haven't thought of Ezio since I sold my Xbox and video games to finance SWAT. Seeing him at EGYcon took me down the memory lane.

On stage, Emma wrapped up a cover for Coldplay. A famous gamer in the gaming community and a singer, Emma was a celebrity on the rise, loved by everybody. She sang covers solo and EGYcon organizers invited her to perform. The crowds cheered and applauded her. Jasmine waved at her. Emma blew some kisses to the crowd and some to Jasmine. After she finished her performance, Emma put down the microphone and got off the stage.

"Daredevil. Daredevil, I came to see you," Emma rushed to greet us.

I felt my cheeks warming up. Given my non existing experience with girls, I felt awkward and didn't know what to answer. I swallowed hard. Jasmine saved the moment and introduced us.

And that's when the fairytale started.

Daredevil was my favorite Marvel character. A blind hero with his eyes covered, he depends on his other senses to find his way around. As a big fan of the TV series, I decided to dress up like him.

And as it happens in movies, Emma, a big fan of the TV series too, hoped to see Daredevil at EGYcon.

Hanging out with people who share your passion and interest is priceless. It felt like going back home to family and old friends. Even if you had no idea who was behind a mask, you were safe. You were not alone. You are among friends you could relate to and who understood you without having to explain yourself. In their company, you were not judged. You didn't have to apologize for who you are, or feel ashamed or awkward that you still watch cartoons, play video games or read comics. For eight full hours, everyone was on the same wavelength, harmoniously co-existed without outsiders staring; without worrying they may look eccentric in the eyes of others, or worse in the eyes of their families. Many families don't comprehend what it meant to be an otaku. They believed cartoons, comics or video games are children's play and a waste of time for adults. For them, engaging in these activities is a sign of immaturity.

Meeting Emma at EGYcon and wearing the costume of Daredevil, her favorite character, was destiny.

"Can you see with your eyes blindfolded," asked Emma.

Of course, I could see, but I wasn't stupid to admit it. I knew that much. "No, I can't see well."

"I will be your eyes for the event."

I liked that.

She grabbed my arm, smiled and winked at Jasmine. Jasmine blinked her green eyes and smiled back.

A music band on stage played SpaceToon songs as we walked away.

"Let's check this out." Emma pointed towards the library where comic artists gathered. We passed VI and Lux from League of Legends who were taking selfies with wolverine, with his sharp razor claws and sideburns. Cameras clicked all around us, and everyone felt like a superhero, and rightfully so. Aren't we all heroes in our own way? Just look at Spiderman clinging to the grass while trying to keep his balance. Darth Vader watched Spiderman and gave him instructions how to move, an epic scene to watch them together.

The sight of Darth Vader teleported me back to the basketball court and reminded me of Mourad, the coach who kicked me out of the team for my obesity. If he could only see me know.

On the walls of the library rooms, comic artists displayed their artwork. Posters, prints and original artwork with characters and scenes from video games hung on the walls. I pretended I could not see them and Emma, amused by this game, laughingly described them to me. A hardcore Marvel fan,

I admit I did not recognize many non-Marvel characters. Several vendors were selling action figures, key chains, comic books, t-shirts and other collectibles. Japanese food served in the food court.

Emma stopped to talk with Asuna from Sword Art Online and a girl I didn't recognize wearing a green skirt and long green hair. Emma explained to me she was Hatsune Miku, a Vocaloid character, the singing voice synthesizer software product.

Video gamers gathered on the other side of the campus where video game tournaments were held. Those who were not playing cheered for their favorite characters, in the game or the ones playing it. We stopped for a game of Mortal Kombat. Emma was a good gamer, but I was a better one. I let her win the game.

Emma and I spent the entire day at the event together until closing time. Time flew, and before we said our goodbyes, I did the dumbest thing in the history of mankind.

"I like you." I told Emma.

"I like you too," she responded.

My heart melted and clouded my judgment. I never felt this warm, fuzzy feeling in my heart before, and I enjoyed it. And with my non existing experience with girls, I didn't know rushing into relationships was a red flag. But I didn't want this fairytale to just end. No matter how I rationalized it to myself, I didn't believe this day just happened, but destiny brought us together. I had bought the ticket to the event a few weeks earlier, and I did not just meet a girl, but by the end of the day I had a girlfriend who told me that she liked me *too*. A fairytale.

We found out we lived close to each other and we rode home together. After the event, we spent two magical weeks together. We met every day and talked on the phone for long hours when we were not together. We went out on dates, played a lot of video games, Bloodborne and Mortal Kombat. I let her win most of the time.

Emma was the first serious relationship in my life, and I jumped full force into it. I fell for her. With my low self-esteem, I was in disbelief that she not only accepted me, but chose me over all the guys who were at EGYcon. No one ever chose me before.

Me.

For the first time in my life I felt confident about myself and actually liked ME. With this self confidence boost, I felt I could do anything.

But of course, when something is too good to be true, it is too good to be true. After two weeks floating on cloud nine I came crashing down. I discovered she was playing me. She already had someone in her life not ready to commit, and she resorted to the oldest trick known; playing hard to get. Flirting with me and going out on dates with me in front of the gamers had been a scheme all along, to grab his attention so he would show his interest in her. And it worked. When he saw us together, he got mad. After two weeks, her plan worked and she left me for him.

I was crushed. Not the best experience in my life, but I am grateful for it, nonetheless. I am grateful for the fairytale I lived in for two weeks. Overall, I had a good time myself for two weeks, despite the hurtful pain she left me in.

I retreated back to my shell. Focused on my studies, school work and SWAT. Because of SWAT and my transformational journey, and with Emma behind my back, amazing things were happening in my life; Personal growth and development beyond my wildest expectations and I savored every moment of it.

*

A DREAM CAME TO LIFE: MY FIRST TALK

"And the spiral of inspiration continues," the event coordinator spoke in the microphone as she paced the stage of Bassily Auditorium. "Our next speaker is an AUC student and the founder of SWAT, Changing People's Lives Through Street Workout. Please help me welcome Abdelrahman Soliman." The audience applauded at the mention of my name. I stood backstage, waited for her to introduce me and retreat offstage before I made my entrance.

At the mention of my name, my heart rate elevated, I feared the audience would hear it pumping all the way in their seats. I had just started my second semester when Peer Advising Leader (PAL) invited me to become a speaker at The TALK, a program initiated by the American University in Cairo to help its freshmen in their transition.

Overwhelmed with anxiety, I squeezed on the microphone with a tight grip to stop my sweaty palm from shaking. To say I was nervous is an understatement. With the adrenaline building inside me, my muscles tensed and I perspired. A burning sensation rushed in my skin and overheated my underarms.

Few seconds is all it takes between the event coordinator exiting the stage and my entrance, but it felt like a lifetime. Nothing prepares you for this moment, no matter how much you rehearse or think you are ready. My throat felt like cardboard and I swigged from the water bottle next to me, gulped for air and filled my lungs with the cool air-conditioned air. Despite how low they kept the temperature on stage, and how I shivered a few minutes ago, the panic and stage fright raised my body temperature. I wiped the sweat beads off my forehead with my palm.

"I can do it. I can do it. I can do it."

I repeated to myself as the adrenaline shot in my veins. I walked in the dark towards the white big letters that stood tall on the ground THE TALK. The orange spotlights reflecting on them. The glossy hardwood floor of the stage was polished and smooth. I worried if the audience heard the noise of the wood squeaking under my feet. Then I worried at the thought of slipping and falling on the polished floor.

"I can do it. I can do it. I can do it."

The lights in the auditorium were off, which made it even more intimidating. Bassily's stage is terrifying. It is the main university auditorium with a capacity of 1255 seats. It is where the main university international conferences and events are held. Equipped with the cutting edge audio-visual devices, it guaranteed transmitting the sound of my fear and anxiety to the audience.

At my sight, the audience applauded and cheered. As I walked toward them, they roared. I heard few familiar voices, but could not see any features, just silhouettes of friends, acquaintances, classmates and many others I did not know. It comforted me that Karim, and Yehia, my partners at SWAT, and Zeyad, sat among the audience. All eyes were fixed on me. I did not want just their eyes, but their ears too. Their full attention. I took center stage, moved away from the orange spotlight, still glowing on the letters THE TALK. In the vastness of the dark auditorium, I felt like standing at the edge of the universe, a feeling that was both fearful and humbling.

As most of my college mates, Maha had never set eyes on me before the school year started, hence clueless of my *"Before"* phase. We sat at the college cafeteria together one day having lunch when she commented on my food choice and quantities I consumed. Not many 18-year-olds are health conscious, especially when it came to their food and diet, and that is how our conversation about weight loss started. I told her I had lost 50 kg. She laughed in disbelief.

"You are joking, right?" She tilted her head to one side, stole quick glances at me, as if trying to imagine how I looked with this excess weight. She shook her head, "No way. Tell me you're making it up."

I pulled my phone out of my pocket, accessed my transformational video on YouTube, played it and handed it over to her. Her eyes popped as she watched. Her gaze travelled in disbelief from the screen to my face to the salad bowl and sugarless black coffee in front of me, and back to the screen.

"Unbelievable," she muttered in awe when the video ended.

Both inspired and amazed, Maha showered me with questions about health, diets, nutrition, weight loss, life styles and challenges. I recounted to her my weight loss journey and answered all her questions, which impressed her even more. She informed me she was a member of the university events committee.

"We are looking for a speaker for our upcoming event." It was me whose eyes popped this time. "You will be a good fit for our talk," she assured me.

Pleasantly surprised by her invitation, and despite my lack of public speaking skills, I immediately agreed without hesitation. I had always wanted to inspire people, and THE TALK would be the perfect opportunity for me to do so; a dream come true. We exchanged phone numbers, and a few days later I received a phone call from the organizers, as promised. They wanted to meet with me first, ask some questions and listen to my story before they made their decision.

I arrived at the meeting cautiously optimistic, but it turned out better than I had anticipated. The organizers listened attentively as I told my story, again. When you have lost 50 kg, everyone wants to hear how you did it, and I never got tired repeating it. On the contrary, repeating it filled me with pride and excitement, as if I'm telling it for the first time; a perpetual reminder of what I had been through. Excitement is contagious, I felt it in the air. Their eyes shined in admiration as they watched the transformational video and heard about my startup to help people lose weight. The impression I made on them exceeded my expectations, and by the end of the meeting they had already made the decision. THE TALK is a go. The dream became a reality, but with it came responsibilities I was not ready for but willing to learn.

I left the office filled with mixed emotions of elation and apprehension. As much as I wanted to do it, I started doubting myself, my readiness and ability to stand in front of an audience and talk to them. My self-confidence, or lack of it, to be precise, hovered over my head as I walked away. By the time I reached the gate, I wanted to turn back and apologize for accepting the task. Tell them I remembered a deadline for an important term paper I had to work on, or I had forgotten about a prior engagement that day with NASA, to circumnavigate the globe in a space shuttle. Thank them for the opportunity and promise to participate in a future event.

As the metro rattled on its tracks towards Maadi, where I was giving a training session, I started compiling the talk in my head. I knew exactly what I wanted to say. I told my story tens of times, maybe even hundred times. The challenge was how to overcome my fears and shyness, stand in front of a life audience and repeat it one more time.

Silence befell in the auditorium. I froze in place for a few seconds, overwhelmed with joy, exhilaration, fear, anxiety, pride, and other fuzzy and warm feelings, and many more scary ones. The seconds felt like hours, like a lifetime. My life time, a journey that led me to this point, to this spot. The moment was mine to savor and cherish. Mine alone. For me, my accomplishments up to this moment were comparable to summiting Everest. Bassily's Auditorium was my Everest. In the nervousness of the moment, I saw the stage camera moving, reminding me the moment is real. Powerful. Intense.

Where is my voice?

The organizers reviewed my speech and I had rehearsed it on the same stage for days, but the allure of life audience was powerful and intimidating. Everything I prepared for and rehearsed evaporated from my head. The microphone still held tight in my sweaty hand. The eyes still staring at me in the dark. Everyone came to hear me talk. I had a message I wanted to deliver to them. It was crucial for me that they listen, but first, I had to find my voice and stop myself from running away.

I had to speak. I could not just stand and stare back at them in the dark.

"I can do it. I can do it. I can do it."

I took a deep breath, raised the microphone to my mouth with a shaky hand and greeted the audience. I had minutes to engage them, to deliver my story which I crafted to be truthful, engaging and interesting. I stood on stage not only to present myself, but also to tell the story of everyone who shared the same experiences, and suffered because of their weight or body image. I wanted the talk to be a force of change, an answer to their uncertainties. I wanted the audience to walk away inspired, motivated, energized, and most importantly hopeful. I wanted to give them one message. "If I made it, so can you."

With the visual aids displayed on the stage screen perched above my head, showing glimpses of my early life, my old me, I talked about how to overcome and solve problems and challenges we face in our lives; using my life journey as an example.

Counting the days and hours to the event was nerve wracking. While anxious to share my experience, I was apprehensive about who really cared to hear the story of a fat boy who lost weight. On the outside, my story sounded like one you have heard a hundred times before. Everyone at some stage in their lives took action to lose weight. But probing into it, it revealed more than just a weight loss success story. I had a vision and a purpose, and finally I had the platform to deliver them. As the countdown to the event started, the self-doubt and insecurities I have worked hard to bury, floated back to the surface. The day before the event, haunted by nightmares of all things that may go wrong, sleep eluded me. It was my first public speaking and I feared people would just walk out, fidget in their seats and fight their boredom by playing with their cellphones.

Under the orange spotlight, I started to talk. My fears melted away and everything came back to me. I opened my heart and spilled it out, and when I finished everyone applauded. The sweetest sound I have ever heard to date. Standing on Bassily's stage was a pivotal moment and memorable experience in my life. Despite being short of 8 minutes, the message I delivered resonated with the audience. After the talk, they walked to me, shook my hand, patted me on the shoulder and congratulated me on my achievement. Until today, people who had attended remember my talk.

THE TALK was one of the best experiences I had in my life and I wished from my heart it made a difference is someone's

ABE SOLYMAN

life.

*

HOW I BECAME A YOUNG ENTREPRENEUR?

I did not expect losing weight would make me so popular. People who knew me were shocked, awed and amazed by the transformation; and of course, intrigued by how I achieved it. I became known as the guy who lost 50 kg. The same guy who, not many years ago, they knew as the boy who weighed 90 kg, but it seemed like a lifetime in between.

And because actions speak louder than words, what I had accomplished was massive, not just in my eyes, but in the eyes of everyone who saw me. Without exaggeration, guys who once humiliated and bullied me, contacted me and asked for my help to lose weight.

"How did you do it?"

"Tell us how can we lose weight?"

They flooded me with questions. For the first time in my life I felt I was of value to others. I had never been in this spot before and I became proud of myself. Them reaching out to me, rewarded me for all the wrong doings and torment they once inflicted on me. In a sense, it was my revenge, even though I had not plotted for it or saw it coming. Only then I understood Frank Sinatra's quote, "The best revenge is massive success."

Revenge is sweet indeed. However, when they came to me asking for advice, I did not hesitate to share with them the knowledge and information I gained on my journey. No doubt the attention flattered me, but I neither sought the attention nor the applause. I found joy in helping people to lead a better life. I did not want anyone to experience what I went through, or suffer because of it.

As the number of people seeking my help increased, the situation became overwhelming. I could not give each my full attention. An alternative to answer their individual questions, I invited them to exercise with me instead. To see me in action. Get a grasp and taste of my new world. Surprisingly, many expressed interest and joined me at the gym. We worked out together, and I gave them tips and advice on how to exercise and what to eat. I even followed up on their diets. Many witnessed progress in a short time. It was then that I realized I wanted to motivate people and help them lose weight. And hence the idea of the transformational videos was born; a spur of the moment decision.

Karim and I created two videos and uploaded them on YouTube; One for losing weight and the other for building muscles. Karim, in contrast to me, was not just slim, but rather skinny. With exercise, he built a lot of muscles. Obviously, I created the weight loss video and Karim created the muscles building one. We also hung out with Yehia and Zeyad. Yehia exercised with us, but he neither needed to lose weight nor cared to build muscles, just fascinated by the whole process and doing epic stuff, like walking on his hands. He had nothing to contribute to the content of the videos, but helped us to make them. Zeyad on the other hand, wasn't interested in exercising, but he hung out with us because he loved our spirit and enjoyed watching our transformation.

At the beginning and at the end, inspiring others was what motivated me. The core message of my transformational video was to show that even obese people can become heroes. "Hey, look at me," I wanted to say, "I am a normal guy with a normal life. I took care of myself and I saw results. And as I managed to change myself and my life, so can you. I am the living proof that no one has an excuse not to try to change their bodies and lives if they wanted to, and succeed."

We recorded the transformational videos and uploaded them on YouTube. At that time, I did not know much about YouTube or how it worked. I just uploaded the videos and dumped them there. What followed exceeded our expectations. Within a few days, the viewership surged. Clueless about the world of YouTube, when I mentioned the number of viewers to people and friends, they were in awe. Apparently transformational videos were among the top videos that reached a wider audience, had the most follow and view, but I did not know it then. For me, I merely wanted to document my journey and wished for some people to watch it and be inspired. Later, I realized the story itself contributed the most to the success of the video. The video delivered an emotional story of a young fat boy who struggled and strived to lose a lot of weight. Viewers connected with me on a personal level.

After the release of the video, more people called me and asked for advice. When the video view reached 60,000 (it eventually reached 200,000) we decided to start SWAT, the business — I was ready to take my experience to the next level, which I did not plan for, but led to by my new discovery and passion to inspire, motivate, guide, help and lead people in their journey of transformation.

Starting the business was another spur of the moment decision. We sat together, the three of us savoring the moment, celebrating the 60,000 views, when the idea to turn this success to our good advantage hit me.

"Let's train people."

Without a second thought, the idea received unanimous approval, "okay."

We needed a place and credibility. The day following our

entrepreneurial decision to start SWAT, I went online and registered with the International Sports Sciences Association (ISSA), and within eight weeks, I became a certified trainer, one of the youngest who received this certification in Egypt. Neither Karim nor Yehia believed in the importance of becoming certified trainers at that time.

Zeyad was elated when he heard the news, and despite we did not include him as a partner since he wasn't interested in our core belief, when we launched SWAT, he offered to help us. He joined SWAT as a team member. It was interesting to see how SWAT changed his life too, as he also went through his own transformation, from someone who didn't care about exercising to becoming one of our trainers, among many other responsibilities he took.

What made this period in my life even more memorable, was that it witnessed the first time I ever talked to a girl, and sustained a relationship for three full days. Three days are a blink of an eye in anyone's life, but for me, they were a big deal. Never in my life before had a girl acknowledged my existence, let alone talked to me. I looked so down on myself — I still do — that until Lucy walked into my life and walked out three days later, I had never thought a girl would be interested enough to talk to me, or to listen to anything I had to say. Lucy and I became good friends and are still in contact till this day. She will always have a special place in my heart. She marked her spot as the first girl in my life who actually liked me.

When I started college, SWAT had been in operation for one month. We officially launched the business in August 2015, with a gentlemen verbal agreement. We were young, exhilarated and enthusiastic to launch our business. Signing legal partnership papers or even a contractual agreement never crossed our minds. When it started, SWAT was not the best business model, but for 15 and 16-year-olds, it was a real success entrepreneurial story. We created a business out of nothing. We just needed a place to direct the influx of people who wanted to exercise with us. We rented the Sadeya training fields to serve as our training grounds; the same grounds where not long ago I practiced Parkour.

Since I had no prior business experience, I negotiated with the owner the worst deal ever. We had agreed to charge LE 25 per person, with a minimum of five people to have access to the place. The owner asked for 60 percent of our gross income. The remaining 40 percent would be divided by the three partners. With a simple calculation, the owner's cut for every person we trained was LE 15. That left LE 10 to be divided among the partners. Thus, for each person we trained, I received LE 3.33 - by 2020 exchange rate, this equals $0.2.

We started with ten trainees. The three of us net gained

LE 100 from each session. We agreed to save the revenues, with which we bought a portable training bar. It did not take us long to realize we had been duped, but failed to renegotiate a better deal. We started looking for other options, exploring the possibilities of using gym facilities for a monthly rent.

Meanwhile we conducted our training sessions at Sadeya, we also visited gyms across town to sell them our idea. If you think marketing new concepts is challenging, imagine what it was like for 15-year-olds asking gym owners to go in business with them for a percentage of the revenues. It goes without saying, no one took us seriously. Many made fun of us, some even laughed in our faces as they showed us the way out.

"Okay dear, we will call you." They never did.

At other gyms, they just kept us waiting and then asked us to leave without even hearing our offer. Some went as far as to tell us the manager was not in, while he walked around. We were ridiculed and turned down in so many different ways, but nothing deterred us from our goal.

In the scorching heat of the summer, after I finished exercising or training at Sadeya, I spent every minute of my day visiting gyms to sell them our concept. I did not understand why they turned us down. We were offering them a zero-risk business opportunity. Not only did they have nothing to lose, but we also offered them a monthly rent to use their facilities at specific times per day. I walked around town with a long list of gyms, with phone numbers and addresses. I visited each one of them, exchanged phone numbers, crossed them off the list, and waited for someone to call me.

Persistence eventually paid off. Finally, we received an offer from a gym in Mohandeseen, called 'The Gym'. Its management agreed to allow us to use their facility for a flat fee of LE 1800 per month, paid in advance. We had been saving our revenues from training at Sadeya. Two months after we started SWAT, we had saved enough money to pay the rent at Mohandeseen, with LE 100 to spare. We were elated. Our concept was selling and we decided to take the risk. In the first month, we covered the rent and made some money.

As the business developed, we adjusted our model again to fit our business approach. Instead of paying rent, we offered gyms a different deal. Use their facilities for a percentage of our profits. A brother of one of my friends opened a CrossFit box in Maadi and he agreed to our deal, for 60 percent of our profits.

Concurrently, Zeyad negotiated an even better deal for us with H2o gym, also located in Mohandessin. We went into a 50/50 partnership agreement. It was the best accomplishment for our business thus far. Within three months after SWAT started, we were operating in two locations in Cairo; Mohandeseen and Maadi, under our terms. From there on, the partnership agreements with the gyms we operated at across town ranged between 50 to 60 percent.

We trained calisthenics, a novelty back then in Egypt. Calisthenics is strength and resistance training. It consists of a group of compound exercises that use one's own body weight as resistance. Calisthenics training requires minimal equipment to build muscles, mostly bars and free weights instead of exercise machines. The sport dates back to ancient Greece and was used for training Alexander the Great's armies and the Spartans.

It is a full body workout. Not only does it drop weight, but also builds and shapes muscles. Designed to increase and improve strength, fitness, flexibility, agility, coordination and balance, Calisthenics workout includes a variety of exercises such as squats, lunges, crunches, dips, pushups, pull ups, board jumps, and even jumping rope. One of the major benefits of Calisthenics is that it reduces the risk of injuries in comparison to weight lifting.

With the expansion of the business, we needed equipment; pull up and dip bars, barbells and dumbbells, because gyms were not equipped for calisthenics training yet. A rough estimate indicated we needed LE 2500. We tried to come up with money, but we couldn't. Both Yehia and Karim were broke.

The only possession of value I owned was my Xbox. It had a more emotional value to me than its material worth.

My Xbox; my lifelong friend and companion. I spent countless hours, sleepless nights playing video games. I became so attached to it and it pained me to depart with it. But I had to. I had a purpose and a mission and I knew I was giving up my video games for a good cause. The other reason I did not hesitate to invest in buying the equipment we needed is because I believed in SWAT and in the business model we created. I had a larger than life vision for it, an investment worthwhile.

I sold the Xbox and the games for a good price of LE3000. We bought the equipment we needed, and put aside some cash for unexpected business expenses. Despite us dividing the profits by three, I was the one who capitalized the business from selling my video games. Later on, as the business developed, Karim paid an equal amount of LE 3000, which we used to buy more equipment. Yehia had no means to finance SWAT back then.

By the time I started college, SWAT operated in two locations; H2o in Mohandeseen and Fit Factory, Crossfit Box in Maadi.

*

THE FALL OF SWAT

For a freshman, college was not an easy ride. The transition from high school overwhelmed me. The protective bubble I lived in with 30 or 40 classmates burst, and with no prior social skills or experience, I found myself like a fish out of water, competing and interacting with thousands of students on campus. At the beginning, I found it hard and intimidating to cope and it took me a while to adjust to my new surroundings. I am not really an introvert, but I had been left out most of my life, and dealing with people had not been my forte. I had to learn how to develop the social skills I lacked from scratch.

In college, I behaved like a kid in a candy store. Curious to learn more and to meet new people, I interned at various students' activities and joined many clubs. I decided to join these clubs for many reasons; to meet new people, connect and learn how to deal and interact with them, and networking. The second important reason I joined was because I wanted to learn more about running a business, the operation and financing, to be able to grow my own business. I did not join with the purpose to have some fun on campus. I had a goal in mind that I wanted to achieve.

I became more involved in the programs they offered, especially the business ones. The world of business intrigued me. I completely related to Albert Einstein's quote, "The more I learn, the more I realize how much I don't know." And thus, I wanted to discover everything about business and how to implement these business practices to grow and develop SWAT. From these clubs I also learned that business is not just delivering a product, but that a product is the end result of the business operation. In other words, using SAWT as an example; SWAT was divided into two divisions; coaching which is basically training people and trying to help them lead a better and healthy life, and the other part is marketing, operation, financing, documentation, and whatever it takes to run a business.

College was a whole new adventure for me. It required my full attention, attendance and participation. In between attending classes, clubs' meetings, and school assignments, my days were overloaded. Not to mention that I studied computer science, nothing to sneeze at either. In addition, I spent two hours every day commuting from home to college, one way, a total of four hours to get to college and back. And with a startup on my plate that also required my full attention and dedication, life got complicated.

I still had the same 24 hours to accomplish everything I needed to, and with my overflowing schedule, juggling my college and work responsibilities became challenging. And while everything that went on in life competed for my attention, the first problem emerged with SWAT. With my limited time, my responsibilities at the company dwindled. I did not have the luxury of time to lead many training sessions and I had to make some adjustments to my training schedule. A decision frowned upon by my partners.

The first two years at college were very stressful. During the day, I attended lectures and meetings at the clubs and participated in their activities. Every day after I finished my classes, I hurried to get to the training sessions on time. I had no car then and I used public transportation, buses, minivans and the underground metro to get to the gym in Maadi, on the other side of town. Back home, which took two more hours on a good day, I had to work on my school assignments and papers, and study for class quizzes and exams. I had no time to scratch my head, and hardly any to sleep. I gave up my social life entirely, which had started to flourish, but I had no time for it either.

College years are the best time in the lives of students, so I have heard. The time to have fun and live freely before life's responsibilities kick in, but I did not have the luxury of this joie de vivre. I did not mind. My vision, message, purpose, mission and goal in life were bigger, and I wanted to learn more about how to reach them. My utmost mission was to help people change, and maybe make money along the way, but the financial gains were not my motivation or driving force.

While my days were loaded, with no time to scratch, Karim, Zeyad and Yehia's lives ran smooth. They lived closer to their colleges, which were not as demanding as mine either. They had more time to dedicate to SWAT and training. Zeyad, despite not being a partner, or perhaps because of that, he was the only one who understood my dilemma, and sympathized with me.

On the other hand, Karim and Yehia started holding grudges against me. They were even vocal about it. They talked behind my back and in my face. They confronted me on several occasions, didn't spare an opportunity to object and criticize me for working less hours than them. With Karim's manipulative and controlling character, always complaining he worked the hardest, training more sessions that I did, and with Yehia chanting along with him, tension started; the first nail in the coffin.

With the pass of time, we stopped seeing eye to eye on SWAT. Our vision for the company's growth and development started to move in different directions. As my knowledge about business operation and marketing grew, I realized we were laying the building blocks for a business, not just training people. If we wanted to grow, we had to understand the business concept, and run the operation as such.

I suggested to them we have to learn how to market the business. We have to document the business process and understand the fundamentals of entrepreneurship. But Karim always objected. Karim, at the beginning and at the end, wanted to control the entire operation, and refused to hear any voice but his own. He ran the business like he was the sole owner. He pushed us all on the sidelines and took absolute control of the operation, treated us like employees not partners. Because of Karim's attitude and behavior, Zeyad left.

Coming from a different business culture, Karim discarded my suggestions and recommendations to grow and develop the business, as unnecessary and a waste of time. He objected to all my requests. He refused to document our income and expenses, with the excuse that we did not have time. I volunteered to keep the books, which infuriated him more and he suggested instead of wasting time doing so, I should spend the time conducting classes.

My plans to market the business hit a brick wall. He did not find marketing necessary, but also a waste of time and money. Instead of spending funds on marketing strategies, he suggested we create a video every year, similar to the transformational videos, and that should take care of our marketing.

Developing a business plan was also of no value from his point of view, and he wouldn't even consider it.

No matter what I suggested, Karim declined, and in return he urged me to train more classes instead. Like a parrot, the answer to all my suggestions was to train more classes as I did before I started college. No other aspect in the business operation mattered to him. Blinded by his unilateral vision for the business, he could not comprehend that implementing business strategies would grow our scale and reach. The busier I got, the more stubborn he became to understand and accept I did not have time to give more classes. He wouldn't understand I had a tight schedule, how demanding my college was or that my college years were a temporary phase in my life. Perhaps he understood all that, but found the perfect excuse to exclude me from the business, which was not only my idea, but one that I have also financed and worked hard to grow and develop.

This ongoing conflict caused the division of the team. Zeyad sided with my views. He understood training is just one of the business components, and the operational steps are as important. He also believed marketing will give us more exposure and agreed we had to explore more channels to grow our reach, create new deals and franchise the operation. Our opportunities to grow were served to us on a gold platter. We had done well so far and with little organizational structure, we could have created a fitness storm. But all this fell on deaf ears. Karim and Yehia had zero interest to hear or explore any of the suggestions and options Zeyad and I proposed. We argued and fought continuously. And since Zeyad was not really a partner, he just couldn't take it anymore and walked away.

One of the biggest lessons I learned from this experience was to always appreciate the people you work with, even if you compensated them well. The moral appreciation means more to them than the financial one. Zeyad received neither from us. He helped us to establish the business and worked hard for us. We neither gave him shares in the business nor compensated him for his time and the effort he exerted to help the business grow and develop. But at the same time, we depended on him entirely. We took him along with us everywhere. He was our fourth hand. He had a full training schedule and never missed a session or complained he was not receiving a salary. He even took a session on his birthday and trained just one person, and expected nothing in return. We simply took him for granted and never once thanked him. Not only that, but we even mistreated and disrespected him, including me at times, and we were upset when he expressed his dismay.

Moreover, Karim did not like most of his opinions and views about the business. So, Zeyad had to succumb to Karim's orders and demands, but he didn't like Karim bossing him around. Tension between them started, but at the end, he still followed Karim's orders. But nothing satisfied Karim, he did not care if he stayed or left, and whenever Zeyad complained, Karim dismissed him by saying, if he did not like it he could leave, which he eventually did. Zeyad believed in us and he helped us out of love. He literally did not want anything out of it, other than to see SWAT grow. He is this kind of person, a loyal, faithful and dedicated friend. He did not deserve to be treated the way we treated him.

By the time Zeyad left, I had managed to get us a new deal in October city and another in Tagamo'e, at the gym on campus. I handled Tagamo'e and became in full charge of it. I managed it my way. But with his obsession to control, Karim's interference in every business decision I made became intolerable, and the conflict between us escalated. In addition, Karim and Yehia kept whining they were working more hours than I did, even though I had a big vision for the business than both combined. But they were blind to see the future I had envisioned for the business. They just saw under their feet.

I created a business and marketing plan despite them, and ran Tagamo'e branch the way I learned business from the clubs I joined in college. Resisting any business innovation strategies, every time I mentioned these plans, Karim put them and me down. Self-centered and arrogant, Karim lived in his own head and believed he was always right. We fought together more than we worked together. The business environment and the time we spent together became stressful and unpleasant. Fortunately, we managed to keep the business disputes between us. It did not reflect on the clients. They were content with our service and the results they were achieving. But obviously, it reflected on my mental health and Zeyad's.

Karim treated the business like it was his baby, alone, ignoring that it also belonged to Yehia and I. He treated us like outsiders helping him run his business, according to his rules and orders without interfering. He expected us to follow his decisions without questions or objections. Not before too long, I came to the conclusion that under no circumstances the business will have a chance to grow the way he handled and controlled it.

*

I AM NOT CLINGY...I SWEAR

Watching SWAT Facebook page grows was like watching your firstborn baby crawling, walking and eventually running and talking. Both mesmerizing and delightful to sit back after a long day at college and at the gym and observe the dynamics on the page when we posted a new photo of the team, or wrote about a transformational story. Savoring our success became my daily fix.

With Docdoc napping on the desk in front of me, and listening to Krewella with my headphones, I scrolled down the messages we received. Responding to each and every message in the SWAT inbox was essential customer service, something we all agreed upon. Elementary business practices.

"I am a swimmer and I want to expand my knowledge and wonder if you offer coach training." A message read. It caught my attention. We don't usually get many of these requests. The message came from Layla. Most of the time, I check the sender's profile, to make sure I am communicating with real people, not fake profiles with a lot of time in their hands, and who wear you out asking irrelevant questions, just for the sake of it.

Layla's account looked authentic. "If you are interested, join one of our classes in Zamalek. I can explain to you the procedures. We can start a training program and if you like it, you can join us as a trainer." I wrote back.

The cat twitched, jolted himself out of his nap and stretched his body. I tossed his fetch mouse across the room, but Docdoc yawned, closed his eyes and fell into deep slumber.

I have always believed in the power of social media and digital marketing, and their influence on the growth of the business, any business. I believed it since the early days of SWAT. It was in the forecast for business. I enjoyed reading the positive comments on my pictures, they certainly boosted my confidence, but I believed the direct interaction with people, especially those who sent us messages was more important. Nonetheless, between the three of us, we took it upon ourselves to respond to the flood of messages we received daily; answering fans' inquiries, providing health tips, offering support and encouragement, and for potential clients, we urged them to join our classes. I liked this responsibility, as I saw it as a valuable experience that will help grow the business. It was luck that Layla's message fell in my hands, and I also saw it as another dimension in which we can grow the business. If we succeeded in helping her become a certified coach, we can add this accomplishment to our company's portfolio. SWAT can also offer coaching workshops and perhaps become affiliated with an international sports entity and become their representatives in Egypt. We could be providing the workshops needed for the various fitness certifications.

Before the class started, Layla walked over to me, with her athletic posture and radiant smile. I recognized her from her Facebook profile picture, which didn't do her just. Much prettier than her photo, I was instantly smitten with her.

The music started and I instructed one of my best classes. Her presence energized me. Perhaps I wanted to impress her, to convince her to join us. I couldn't wait for the class to end to get a chance to talk with her. When the music faded, and then stopped; announcing the end of the training session, I wanted to run out of the exercise room before the participants trapped me with their usual questions and after class chitchat. They surrounded me, and I couldn't avoid them. My eyes searched for her. She stood out in the crowd, sweat beads on her forehead, flushed red face and out of breath, but looked content, like everyone in the class, well almost everyone. She wiped her face with a towel and waited patiently until I excused myself. We walked together to the gym cafeteria. She complimented me, saying it was the best class she ever attended and was interested to learn more. Music to my ears.

It had been two years since my short-lived fairy tale with Emma, during which I had few relations. Nonetheless, they were all effective lessons. They contributed to my growth as a person. I learned from my mistakes and moved on.

We sat in the cafeteria. I ordered my usual black coffee and she just sipped from her water bottle. As the new classes started, the crowd thinned out and we talked. For a couple of hours, she had my full attention. It felt good talking with Layla because she was an athlete herself and understood my passion for sports. I explained to her the procedures to become a certified instructor and promised to mentor and teach her everything she needed to know.

We met almost every day for the following two weeks. I really wanted her to join SWAT, and for that, I did my best to prepare her to become a SWAT coach and join our small family. I privately tutored her and shared with her the material I collected over the years and the extensive knowledge I possessed. I explained to her in detail everything I knew about exercising and nutrition. It became obvious I made up excuses to meet up with her to exercise, and to spend longer time together, with the excuse to review and study the material that I gave her. She didn't object. In fact, she enjoyed the time we spent together, always relaxed, content and never in a hurry to leave.

Two weeks after we met, I told her I liked her, and that I

would like to see how the relationship developed. She thought it was sweet, most probably she had expected it, and said she liked me too. Layla appeared in my life at the time when signs of strain in the business relationship with Karim and Yehia had surfaced. Having her in my life during this time was a blessing, a breath of fresh air that helped me cope during this hard time.

Haunted by the demons of my other life, I walked into the relationship carrying the same baggage that I had never been able to rid myself off. Insecurities. Doubts. Obsession. Low self-esteem. Incompetence. And many other negative traits I collected over the years. I had no self worth and as I looked down on myself, I questioned why Layla chose me over everyone else. Not to mention Emma's ghost didn't leave me in peace either. I had thought I healed from the hurt she caused me, but apparently, I had not. I wondered if Layla was using me too, and if she would dump me like Emma did, once she had no use for me anymore. Overwhelmed with these insecurities, I worried and feared I would wake up one day and find Layla gone too.

As a result of my insecurities, I became clingy, nagging and possessive. I called her and wanted to be with her all the time. I demanded her full time and attention. I wanted her to call me every day and pushed her to go out on dates, and she was not the type who liked to go out a lot. I didn't give her enough space to breath, and choked life out of our relationship.

My actions and behaviors backfired. Layla started to lie to me, go out with her friends behind my back, turn her phone off so I can't reach her, tell me she was staying home and go out to the movies with her friends. It bothered me a lot. The more she withdrew, the more obsessive I became.

And it was not a matter of if, this relationship would end, but when....

*

Business partners can make or break the business. If I had any doubts left in my mind about how toxic Karim was, his actions confirmed it. I became aware how he took advantage of me all these years, and continued to do so, until the end. While I considered him my best friend, he treated me like a puppy. He took me for granted, like Zeyad, and abused me the same way he abused him. This realization came as an epiphany, a wakeup call, but I decided I won't quit. I had a message for people, which was important for me to deliver. This message kept me going, and made me tolerate Karim's abuse. I had already helped more than one hundred people to lose weight and change their lives. My purpose and mission were more important to me than Karim's attitudes and behavior. I had to deliver the message to people who counted on me. And if Karim stood in my way, I was ready to run him over and continue on my path. Despite our conflicts, I made an effort to put up with him, but the conflicts and abuse kept escalating. As the tension grew, deep inside I knew the spiral downfall had started, but I ignored the signs, and hoped a miracle would knock some sense into Karim's mind.

Then the day came, Karim and Yehia summoned me for a meeting. I anticipated the outcome, not that I had a crystal ball, but the events in the past few months had built up to that meeting. Yet deep in my heart, I hoped they had finally come to their senses and wanted to talk about the growth of the business. Ironically, the culmination was far from that.

We met in the shooting club, our meeting's headquarters. Without wasting time to sugarcoat the words, Karim bluntly told me they do not want me with them anymore, that I do not deserve to be a partner because they train more classes than I did. Based on that, Karim continued, we cannot be equal partners. Yehia sat there nodding his head, affirming Karim's words. I suggested if they saw I was not giving as much time to the training as they did, despite my other responsibilities, they can decrease my shares in the business. At this stage of the business, we had written and signed a contract we drafted ourselves, not really a legal document, but what the minds of 16-years-olds could come up with. Had the business developed and grown, we definitely would have signed a proper contract.

They refused the option to decrease my shares.

"We want you out," they insisted. "We want you out of the picture completely."

Despite I saw it coming, it still stunned me to hear them kicking me out. Until the last minute, I believed they wanted to reconcile our differences. I begged and I pleaded to stay. I had a bigger mission and purpose. I asked them not to deprive me from what I wanted to do, from working towards my goal. Nothing I said deterred them. They had made up their minds and insisted on kicking me out.

Out.

The brief meeting with Karim and Yehia came like a punch under the belt. At loss of words, and numbed with shock and disbelief, I walked away. As I fought the tears, I felt a lump in my throat. I couldn't swallow, let alone breath. My partners kicked me out of the business; my brainchild, the one I had worked around the clock to develop and grow; the business I sacrificed my social life and life in college for; the business I sold my video games to finance when we started, and sold my mother's vacuum cleaner when we needed cash to buy a camera.

I have no recollection of how I returned home. Back in

my dark hole, I experienced a panic attack for the first time. At first, I didn't comprehend what went on, the shortness of breath, the chest pain, the racing heart and dizziness. I thought I was dying, but I did not. Instead, the wrath inside me took over. And just like Dr. Bruce Banner, I might have turned into a Hulk. For all I know, I lost control over myself, and started pounding and punching the wall. I might have screamed my heart out too. Docdoc ran in fear and lunged to the top of the cupboard, but as I started banging it too, the poor cat flew in the air and took shelter under the bed.

Bang. Bang. Bang. I didn't stop until I smashed the door of the cupboard.

My anger was not just because they took away my business or wounded my soul. They stole my purpose in life from me. And that's what nearly killed me.

The straw that broke the camel's back came one week after Karim and Yehia kicked me out of SWAT. I received a phone call from Layla. She wanted to meet and talk. When a girlfriend calls you to meet and talk, make no mistake, it's a neon sign flashing "Problem Alert."

As we drove around in my black Mitsubishi, she spilled it out.

"Frankly, I feel I am the one wearing the pants in this relationship, and that's not what I want. Look at you. You need to man up. I can't go on in this kind of relationship anymore."

Layla was a smart girl whom I liked a lot. Her bluntness both stunned and disturbed me. Layla didn't break up with me because of my expulsion from SWAT, but the breakup obviously came as a consequence of my irrational behavior following it. Because of the way I behaved in the relationship, the breakup was inevitable. Leaving SWAT just expedited it.

The hurt and despair that followed my expulsion augmented my negative character traits. My controlling, dependence, clinginess, obsessiveness escalated after my episode with Karim and Yehia and became unbearable to Layla. I dumped all my baggage on her, and demanded her full time and attention. I needed her to pamper my wounded ego. Perhaps in a healthier relationship with a solid foundation and mutual understanding, I might have found with her what I was looking for, but in our short bumpy relationship, my attitude and behavior repelled her.

In short, she discovered in me someone different from the image she drew of me when we first met. "When I first met you, you gave me the impression that you are a macho guy. You're an A student and had a business at 19. I believed you were in control of yourself and your life. That's why I liked you. But not this. I cannot continue with you."

"Please don't leave me now. Let's try again. I promise I will change."

I begged. I pleaded. Layla was adamant to split up.

"No. No. No. This has to end, now. I am done."

She repeated the classical line of how we can stay friends, which of course never happens, even to the best of romantic relations.

And she walked out of the car and my life. As I watched her fade in the crowd, my heart pounded and my chest ached. I couldn't breathe and the bitter taste of bile in my mouth nauseated me. I perspired profusely as my trembling fingers tingled. I almost blacked out. I became familiar with the symptoms of panic attacks, as it seems they were all I have been experiencing lately. I took a deep breath and woke up from my trance with the cars beeping around me to clear the intersection I had blocked.

I drove aimlessly. Lindsay Stirling played in the background. I turned it off. Last thing I wanted to hear was Shatter Me, totally inappropriate and too cliche for the situation. I couldn't believe how my world had crumbled and fell apart in front of my eyes, demolished one brick at a time. Everything I worked hard to accomplish in the past four years came to an end in a blink of an eye. Mind boggling how not too long ago, I led a perfect life, or so I believed. I had a business and a girlfriend.

I made some money and most important, I did something I loved, through which I delivered a message of hope to people. In brief, I had everything I dreamed of having. Suddenly, everything vanished. Gone.

Layla, with my help, had worked for SWAT for six months after my departure from the company. The irony! What bothered me more than watching her go and how my life shattered in front of my eyes, was that Layla had left me for the same reasons like her predecessors, in the last two years. With her, I repeated the same mistakes that ended my previous relations. This meant I did not learn anything from them. I was still the same scared and insecure person, which meant I had not grown. In fact, I was stuck in the same mindset that I have strived for the past three years to change. I haven't advanced or moved a step forward even though I assumed I did.

Layla pointed out to me the insecurities I thought I had conquered. The relationship had to end dramatically for me to realize that. This truth agonized me. Another wakeup call that made me realize that the insecurities I had harbored when I was obese still lingered there. I changed my body, but my mind stayed the same. I lived in a skinny body but with the same mentality of the fat person I lived with all my life. My insecurities and lack of self-confidence propelled my fears that she would leave me. As I always looked down on myself, I did not feel my worth, and questioned why she even looked at me. I couldn't see anything of value in me for her to see. Because of mclinging and nagging, she felt she wore the pants in the relationship. She did not like these reversed roles and walked away. I don't blame her.

FALLING DOWN THE SLIPPERY SLOPE

Losing the business and the girlfriend came like a punch in my face, a really hard one. It knocked me off my feet. The following few days after Layla walked out of my life were erased from my memory, as if I had been in a coma. When I came back from the land of nowhere, I started doubting everything I worked hard for and achieved. It felt like I had been living in a big lie; a lie I created and believed. It felt like nothing was real anymore. My life was an illusion, or a delusion of reality.

I felt lonely and unloved. And with both my best friends and girlfriend abandoning me, I feared I will never be loved again in my life. The negative thoughts and emotions surfaced and took control over me. Despite my bleeding wounds, I focused on my studies and I exercised vigorously. They became my last resort. My escape. The angrier I got, the more vigorously I exercised. Not before too long I paid the price. In another unfortunate incident, I over-worked out, didn't follow the safety rules, and I snapped my back. The back injury was the last nail in the coffin.

I stopped exercising because of my back injury, a disaster in itself. Confined once again at home, with no exercise, no video games, tons of food in front of me, and my failed business and relationship, I forgot everything I had worked so hard for. I let the beast out of its cage. Before I knew it, weight crawled back.

Until that point, I had been living on 1200 calories per day for four years, in addition to working out for two or three hours per day. The hardcore life I lived couldn't stand in the face of the dire times I was going through. With the first real test, the shortcomings of my diet and lifestyle emerged. The barricades and fortifications I had been building to protect me collapsed.

In his speech titled "Getting Unstuck," motivational speaker Les Brown said, "Everybody can be positive when they have good health, and they have their bills paid and positive relationships. Everybody can be positive then. Everybody can have a sense of vision then. The true challenge of growth, mentally, spiritually and emotionally comes when you get knocked down."

And boy, was I knocked down? Les Brown's quote made perfect sense to me. It described what I went through. As long as I was in control, I had a positive outlook on life. Once I faced challenges beyond my control, the mental energy was sucked out of me, and I gave in to my circumstances.

Broken, emotionally and physically - just a cliche here, my back was injured, but not broken - I sat in bed, could hardly move. Food became my solace. I ate non-stop, as if punishing myself with food. I would order two large pizzas and devour them to the last bite, without processing my actions. When I finished them, I would still be hungry, and order another take-out or eat half a gallon of ice-cream. With a void in my soul deeper than the black hole, no amount of food I ate satisfied me. No amount of food could fill up this void.

Within two months after I stopped exercising, I gained 30 kg, an average of 3.75 kg/week. Let this sink in. To gain this much weight in such a short span of time showed how vulnerable I became. With some calculations, translating this weight gain into calories means I devoured between 5,000 to 6,000 calories per day.

In a duration of three months, I lost my business, my girlfriend, my shape and the people I helped to lose weight. I have to admit, food calmed me down, just like the old days. And with nothing else in my life to look forward to, I ate and studied.

You might ask how all this affected my studies. Well, throughout my life, even when everything else fell apart, I never lost focus on studying. Even when I went through the lowest points of my life, and despite how much I fumbled, I studied hard and was always an A student. I sustained my academic excellence in school and later in college.

With my meager options and opportunities, I had nothing else to do but study; until I die.

*

RISE OF THE PHOENIX

Food, my drug of choice, didn't disappoint me. When everyone abandoned me, my loyal lifelong companion stood by my side. Once again, it prevailed and promised to get me through this tough time. And sure enough, it delivered. Just like any other drug, it calmed me down, altered my perception of reality and soothed my injured soul. Devouring obscene amounts of foods helped me to cope with the emotional shock, grief and pain caused by the trauma, and to overcome the despair, depression and anxiety associated with it. I survived. Regretfully, I paid a high price. I watched my weight soar in two months, at an average rate of 3.75 kg/week, and I didn't care. The food sedated and numbed me, and that is all it mattered. Under its influence, I fell into a deep unconscious state, almost a self-induced coma.

It took three weeks for the initial emotional shock to subside, and to wake up from the self-induced coma food put me in. When I floated back to the surface, damage was already done. I put the brakes on, and reduced my calorie intake to human consumptions, but my weight didn't drop. Reducing the calories helped me not to gain more weight. I maintained the 30 kg gain, and I didn't give a damn. I no longer cared about my body shape, or to follow a food plan.

My back healed in seven months, and I started to train again, to reverse the damage. This time without following food plans, for I had no mental energy to diet anymore. I did not care to eat healthy or to drop my calories intake. I could not look at a bowl of salad or eat healthy calories controlled meals. You may call me a loser or a failure, but in reality, I had depleted the power to do it all over again. I had spent four years working hard to stay in shape, looking after myself and playing it by the book. I lost everything I worked hard for in just two months. No way I was going to do it again. Not only I had no energy, but also no desire, will power or interest to travel this road again. Needless to say, I did not lose not one iota of body weight.

I spent two years in a dark abyss. Despite my exercise, my weight didn't budge a bit. The first year was the hardest, because mentally I was totally off balance. I collected myself after a year, and started to work on changing my mind set, again. To understand why I made the same mistakes again.

I stumbled into a YouTube channel called Improvement Pill, and it introduced me to 'mindset'. The concept of mindset intrigued me. And with my inquisitive mind, I started reading more about it. While learning about mindset, its meaning, why it matters and how it can be changed, I also discovered my passion for reading. I bought my first book, The Subtle Art of

Not Giving a F***, by Mark Manson. One book led to the other. I read the Compound Effect, by Darren Hardy; Shoe Dog, by Phil Knight; Unlimited Power, by Tony Robbins; Success is a State of Mind, by Les Brown, Mark Victor Hansen and Deepak Chopra, to mention a few. Every book opened my mind in a new dimension. I gained more knowledge about myself and the world around me. This knowledge became a powerful tool in my second journey of transformation, the emotional and spiritual one. I realized my first journey was all about physical changes. I learned from these books that a person has to grow in three dimensions, mentally, emotionally and spiritually, and I lacked all three. That's why I collapsed at the first challenge I encountered. My mindset was not prepared for real life experiences.

In his book, The Power of Habit: Why We Do What We Do in Life and Business, Charles Duhigg talked about the experiments conducted to show willpower, and how it is like a mobile battery. According to Duhigg, our willpower has a storage limit. If we keep depleting it, we will eventually drain it, just like a battery. And that's when we start making bad decisions. That's exactly what happened to me. The effort I exerted to eat 1200 calories per day, while fighting hunger and exercising excessively, depleted me. Fighting the fatigue and exhaustion, caused by my lifestyle, school work, and excessive exercise, drained me. I had no juice left in me to continue the fight. Even the Energizer Bunny could not have sustained this life.

Thus, when I encountered a downfall in my life and I felt I lost my sense of purpose, I fell into a depression that sucked my willpower. Training and following a healthy lifestyle were no longer a priority. I had to survive on the little willpower left in me, barely enough to exercise. I slowed down on my workout. And once I lost my purpose, I also messed up my food plan. I felt I had no need to follow it anymore. Before knowing it, I retreated back to my old habits.

As I read more books, I recognized the mistakes I made and why I ended up doing them. The most interesting book I read was Fat Loss Forever, by Layne Norton and Peter Baker. This book helped me understand everything I wanted to know. Why did I gain weight so fast? Why does every diet work? How weight gain and loss is all about lifestyle and willpower? With this epiphany, I understood that achieving results was a long-term game, not a short term one. No matter how fast we think we can lose weight. No matter how strong we think we are, we are in fact weak. Without changing the environment and becoming more friendly towards our lifestyle, the harder it gets, and we will fall back again someday. We will lose the battle, because it is an endless war. It is important to understand and accept the concept that losing weight is an endless war. Sometimes we win and sometimes we lose. Until they find a magic pill that can change our genes, we will have to keep fighting. This is a fact.

All marketers know it but they do not want to admit it. That is the bad news.

The good news is that working out five hours per day and eating a calorie-constrained meal is not the only solution to lose weight. It is just the short-term solution. There is also a long-term solution that will not only achieve the results we desire, but will also change our lifestyle entirely, to a new one.

After this discovery, I decided to do a second transformation, that will also include a mental, emotional and spiritual transformation in addition to the physical one. To accomplish that, I chose the long-term solution. I have already embarked on the new journey of transformation, which I estimate may take me up to three years, but it is going to be worth it, as I will tailor it to suit my lifestyle, to enable me to live a normal life.

On this journey, I will consume 2500 calories per day instead of 1200 calories. I will have a deficit of 200-300 calories. Translating this into facts; if I decrease my intake by 200-300 calories per day, I can lose a kilo every month. It's not hard to lose 200-300 calories per day; it is equal to a moderate walk for an hour. I am tired of dieting and food deprivation. Tired of eating less calories, and counting calories. Tired of old diets and trying new ones. Tired of spending hours at the gym every day and training endlessly. Tired of feeling guilt every time I derail from an eating or excessive plan. My inability and lack of desire to continue on this path was the turning point for me. I will take control of myself and strive for a similar outcome, one traveled on a different path, that's all.

After two years of self-discovery, I realized my purpose is still alive inside me, like a burning flame. It didn't die when I left SWAT. From the ashes of despair, pain, suffering and failure, I will rise again. My purpose will not die, even after I am gone because I will work hard to instill it in the hearts and minds of those who are suffering, like I once did. After I left SWAT, my purpose emerged in a different form, not only to help people lose weight, but also to inspire them and bring them hope. I want to show people that there is a better tomorrow. This is my bigger purpose. It has always been there when I started SWAT, but the purpose wasn't clear enough in my mind yet. I had to fail, and fail one more time to see it clearly.

It took me two years of doubts and failures to realize my new goal in life. I want to impact people's lives on more levels than before. I want to talk to people. I want to motivate and become a source of inspiration to them. Perhaps I will become a motivational speaker one day to accomplish that.

*

KARMA, IS THAT YOU?

It took me short of two years to come out of this abyss. Not sure if it was divine justice, karma, or whatever name you want to label it, but during my healing journey from the emotional trauma and physical injury, SWAT was dying. It took exactly the same duration of time for SWAT to close down as it took me to heal, after they expelled me from the company. It broke my heart to see it gone, but it was an inevitable ending for a company that lacked vision and management.

With Karim's shortsighted vision - or lack of it - it became challenging for him and Yehia to run and manage the business in all locations. The growth of the operation exposed the lack of his entrepreneurial and managerial skills. He led a business bigger than his capabilities, despite him believing otherwise. Whether they admitted it or not, Zeyad and I were keeping the business in balance. After we left, no matter who they hired to run the business, at the end of the day, they were employees. No one had the heart and the vision Zeyad and I had.

Karim, as stubborn as always, took the business for granted, didn't waste time or effort to develop it or understand the aspects of management. As More gyms opened and offered the same programs we did, people faded out from SWAT. No new members joined and the number of recurrent members decreased. And with no records kept, they didn't even know how to get in touch with the previous members to offer them new deals. And because Karim loved to play the victim, he blamed the decline of the business on everything else other than the real reason; his incompetence to run it. He neither solved any problems nor suggested solutions, and the numbers kept declining.

SAWT on Campus, the one I managed alone, closed down first. October branch followed. They divided their responsibilities between Maadi and Mohandessen, but with their zero marketing, while other gyms were flourishing, their business kept declining. Within 18 months after they kicked me out, SWAT closed. Regretfully, it's no longer on the map, a painful ending for a business that had started with so much potential and opportunities ahead to take the market by storm. A bad ending for Karim too. If he had just listened from the beginning, we could have all been ahead of the curve today. Karim decided to leave the business altogether. Yehia took over the business and changed the name to RiseFitness. As of the writing of this book, RiseFitness has one branch in October city, and Yehia became its sole owner. Hopefully, he can make our dream come true one day, fingers crossed.

Despite the pain of watching my baby die in front of my eyes and not being able to revive it, I must admit that the rise and fall of SWAT was an entrepreneurial experience I am very grateful for. Without it, I would have never understood my main purpose. I would not have written this book, and I would not have done many of the things I have accomplished so far in my life.

Karim and I remain friends to this day. I just had to set boundaries between us. Like other relationships people build in their lives, childhood friendships and business partners can also turn toxic, and one must let go. Karim is my lifelong buddy. We share many memories of school, life and business. I am grateful I met him, but cutting the bond was essential, for me to be able to maintain my mental and emotional health.

*

PART THREE
Social Media

DON'T JUDGE PEOPLE BY THEIR SOCIAL MEDIA COVER.

Sitting in bed, after a hard working day at the office and at the gym, I scroll through my newsfeed and watch the whitened teeth, and perfect smiles and bodies. With my busy work schedule I no longer have the luxury to spend four hours at the gym every day as I used to. Watching photos and videos of people with amazing figures and wonderful lives after a bad training day or a day I ate unhealthy, devastates me. Reading about how they succeeded in what I had failed at leaves me feeling depressed and intimidated, even if my day was normal and good. But what really is normal? Normal became so distorted by the unrealistic standards and expectations of social media.

In today's world, there is no escape from social media. We are continuously bombarded by photos, videos and news from friends, family members, work colleagues and celebrities. It is partially our fault because we even follow accounts of people we do not know, simply to watch what they do. No one forces us to do so, but curiosity is just human nature. People love to watch the lives of others, and subconsciously compare it to theirs. Big companies and brand names have researched, studied, analyzed and published reports about consumerism. They have discovered our psychologies before we even knew what was going on. With their understanding of the power of social media and its impact on its users, and with the exorbitant amounts of money paid to promote various brands, influencers were born, to add to the misery of their followers. Despite its soaring popularity, browsing through the various social media platforms is becoming an unpleasant experience for many users, including myself.

No matter your age, gender, profession, social or educational background, there are enough influencers who will remind you of what you are not. These influencers are people like you and me, yet they are not. It is important to note that not all influencers get paid by brand companies. Some are their own brand, and others just love to stay in the spotlight. They do it for publicity and show off. They love the attention and become addicted to likes and shares.

Paid or unpaid influencers offer us unsolicited advice. They tell and show us every detail of their super amazing flawless lives, even if in reality their lives are bland and colorless. They perpetually remind us of our shortcomings and failures. Infiltrating our lives at any given moment of the day or night, they constantly remind us we are not beautiful enough, rich enough, cool enough, amazing enough, fashionable enough, skinny enough, enjoying life enough, not loved enough, our teeth are not white enough. We despise them despite our obsession with them and we welcome them into our lives with opened arms.

We tend to forget while some influencers are paid six figures by brand companies, and many others are striving to show up on the radar of these companies, we are not. While we struggle with our jobs, studies, families, and relationships, these influencers work hard to stay in shape and to look their best. They hire personal trainers, nutritionists, stylists, make-up artists and an army of people behind the cameras to help them shine and sparkle in front of our eyes. Influencing us is their job, and in the competitive world of social media, the harder they work to stay in the frontlines, the more we feel like failures and losers. No matter what facts we know about their fictitious and often superficial lives, we simply cannot help not to compare ourselves with them, and our lives with theirs. With the glamour of their lives, we tend to forget they too have shortcomings, and neither them nor their lives are perfect, just like the rest of us. Looking their best is their job, and they just have to excel in it.

UNFAIR AND UNREALISTIC COMPARISONS

Unfortunately, it is not only the influencers we compare ourselves and our lives with, but on a smaller scale, our friends, family members and work colleagues also become our rivals. Their photos fill us with inferior feelings. It does not matter that some have hired professional photographs or took hundreds of pictures until they found the perfect one to share, after they even airbrushed it with all the new apps designed for this particular reason. Knowing all that, they still intimidate us.

Social media has distorted the perception of reality in the minds of many, including myself. Unlike me, many are delusional of its effect, or unaware of it. Consciously, I am aware of its effect, subconsciously I have already walked the plank and fell into its clutches. How could I not? I am only human. The sad truth is we are all addicted to it, just on different levels.

Social media is a big part of my life. Consumed by it on a daily basis, triggers many undesired feelings inside me. Regretfully, I am unable to break away from it as part of my job involves working on and with its various platforms. In a way, I am like a chef who cannot stay away from the kitchen, even if he's allergic to the vapors of the food he's preparing. Actually, I am even worse than the chef who can quit the kitchen and walk away from its vapors, because unfortunately in today's wired world, I cannot quit my job.

The vast majority of people, influencers included, do not show their vulnerability. They do not share stories when they are in a bad mood or going through rough times. When an influencer was asked how she keeps smiling, looks happy, and her videos are filled with positive energy and laughter all the time, she answered, "The days I am feeling down or not in a good mood, I am not on social media. You only see the best of me. I never talk about my frequent visits to my psychiatrist whom I have been visiting for the past seven years." Quite a humbling answer that reminds us that not everything that glitters is gold. Social media users tend to forget that. Thus, they compare their lives with the lives of others, which becomes quite toxic for them.

I have to admit, it did not bother me as much until after my downfall. As my life spiraled down, I strayed from the course I strived for years to follow. I lost everything I persevered to accomplish. Inevitably, the weight crawled back. With my failure to control my weight gain and to get back on track, and with the new challenges I faced while unsuccessfully trying to lift myself up, I drowned in my misery. Watching success stories of others on social media belittled me and pushed me deeper into an abyss of sorrow. Social media simply amplified the impact of my downfall, my failure.

The more I slipped back into my old patterns, the more weight I gained. As it has gotten harder to lose weight, I became more intimidated by the photos and videos of people who seemed to be in control of their lives, even though I knew in reality they were not. No one stands in front of the mirror and says, I look awful today. I have gained five pounds, let me take a picture and share it with the world. People only share their most attractive pictures, when they were looking good in the summer, with the six pack abs they worked hard all winter to build.

Nonetheless, their photos with sculpted abs, biceps and six pack trigger jealousy inside me. They show a video snippet of their workout, and I know the strenuous daily workout it takes to reach this body shape. They share photos of their colorful healthy meals to impress us. And I know they are starving themselves, counting their calories to have the bodies they show to the world.

UNACHIEVABLE STANDARDS

Surviving social media and living a normal life despite it, is becoming my new challenge. I am confident it is not mine alone. Many people feel the same way. They just do not share their thoughts publicly in fear of blame for being jealous, envious, or wishing ill on others. I have worked out strenuously, starved and deprived myself from food items I love for four years to achieve the socially accepted body image. Even though I have no intention to continue living this way for the rest of my life, nonetheless, when I watch people's photos on social media, I still cannot help not to compare myself to them. My failure with their success. My chubby body with their shaped ones.

Even after a good day at the gym, watching photos and videos of people exercising harder than I did put me down. So, you can only imagine the amount of failure and frustration I feel on a day I could not meet my training goals, because of exhaustion, not in an exercise mood, or any other reason. On these days, I feel I failed as a human being, even though it was just another normal day in my life, and it is okay not to give 100 percent all the time, not even 90 percent or less. It is okay. Really. Even though social media made us believe that we need to give more than 100 percent to belong to the ranks of achievers.

This is the real problem. Social media raised the bar, put high standards and expectations and created a superficial competitive world that often paralyzes and hinders people from reaching their potentials. What we see on its various platforms is unrealistic. It is impossible for the higher percentage of people to live a normal life by these standards. People become motivated to excel to meet the expectations of others, only not to be judged by them. Many strive to become who others want them to be, rather than who they want to be. As they try to achieve these standards and fail, they feel inadequate and imperfect, and may fall into depression.

Thus, it is important to be aware of how social media can influence our thoughts and behaviors. It is okay not to have a six pack, or not to eat healthy all the time. By all means, this is not an invitation to overeat or live a sedentary life. What I mean here, it is okay to eat pizza and cookies if you crave them. It is not the end of the world. Eating them does not make you a loser or a failure. You are just a human being. And as humans, our lives are filled with failures along our successes. Even the most successful achievers have failed, more than once. What we see on social media and in the news are their moments of success that they show us. They do not share with us the tens or hundred times they failed before they reached this success.

It is okay not to strive for or seek perfection all the time. While practice makes perfect, seeking perfection is often toxic. It reminds us that we can not. But what if we really can not do this, or this, or that. We all have the abilities to excel in certain fields, and by practicing hard we achieve results. But not everyone should become an athlete or a painter or a dancer, or a scientist unless they have the interest and desire, and not merely to fulfill someone else's dreams or expectations.

No one is judged if they stopped painting, writing, playing music or if they dropped out of medical school, because they did not find it fulfilling, or for whatever reason they decided not to accomplish what they have started. Society is more forgiving. It does not even pay attention to them. On the other hand, the same society does not waste a chance to label and judge someone who is out of shape, or dressed differently. It is very sad.

Not everyone is a scientist. Not everyone is a model, athlete or a movie star either. And we cannot live by their standards or the life they live. While we have nine to five jobs, for these pop culture celebrities, the acting, modeling or winning games is their job, profession and career. Staying in shape and looking good is their investment in their profession, just like the rest of us attending a seminar or a workshop to improve the client/corporate relationship. For them, looking good and staying in shape on stage, runway, the red carpet, or the field is a requisite for their jobs. But even these celebrities do not diet, pump iron or look healthy and fashionable all year round, around the clock. Yet we don't call them failures. They look perfect when they want us to see them as such, in real life or on social media platforms. The rest of the time, they are just like us.

Look at Hollywood stars. Their photos on magazine covers, in movies and on social media don't present who they really are. When they are caught on camera on vacations or off movie sets, some of them are barely recognizable. Paparazzi make more money selling pictures of celebrities carrying on with their daily normal lives than on the red carpets. Despite them invading their private lives, paparazzi humanized these celebrities in our eyes. We see them overweight, disheveled, dressed in shabby clothes, carrying their babies with runny noses, changing their diapers, pushing their strollers, and eating junk food just like the rest of us. None of this makes them losers or failures in our eyes.

BAD DAYS HAPPEN TO GOOD PEOPLE

It is important to realize and accept that not all days are equal. Good days and bad days are part of life. Some days you will be the best person out there, have the best exercise, eat the healthiest food and stay within the number of calories on your eating plan. Other days you will be the exact opposite, and you will not be the best person out there; not even close. This does not mean you are bad, loser, or failure. It is just another variable. It is what defines you as a human being.

What makes a difference though is how you cope with these "not so good" days. Thus, it is crucial to learn to identify the patterns when these days hit you. Do not dwell on them and understand that they will pass, like any storm. Make a mental note on these days to try harder to do better the following day. Even then, if you did not achieve the goal you set for yourself, do not despair. Acknowledge you have tried, and this in itself is worth a lot. Celebrate every time you try harder, even if you slip, instead of hitting yourself on the head for failing to live up to the standards of others. It is important to be kind to yourself.

Hug yourself and give it a pat on the shoulder. Keep accomplishing small wins that eventually lead to big success. Keep shedding small layers of fat, the grams add up, and down the road you will inevitably see results.

Once you break the barrier of perfection, you will accept yourself as a human being and embrace your shortcomings. You will like your reflection in the mirror, instead of standing in front of it despising your image and fantasizing about cutting your body fat off. Once you reconcile self-acceptance, you can improve and grow without beating yourself up.

I had to go a full circle to understand that I do not have to be in my best shape every day, and it is okay to be out of shape sometimes. I came not only to realize, but also to accept there are ups and downs, and as everything else in life, weight and staying in shape is never constant, but also a variable. My fall and the multiple failing attempts, to rise up to the standards I had once lived by, was a revelation. It opened my eyes to another myth, another perspective about weight gain and loss.

In the book "Fat Loss Forever: How to Lose Fat and Keep it Off" by Layne Norton and Peter Baker, the authors explain that 90 percent of people achieve great results at losing weight. Most people manage to lose the weight they were targeting; 20 kg, 30 kg or even more. The saddest part though is that more than 85 percent of these people gain back the weight. Some may even gain more weight than before they started their weight loss journey.

Against the belief of many, losing weight is the easiest part of the journey, even though it is hard and challenging, and many give up halfway. But once people overcome the physical, psychological or emotional hurdles, push themselves and embark on the journey, decrease their food intake and exercise regularly, they eventually achieve the desired results. There is no art in it.

However, there is more perspective to weight loss than just the process of losing it. Once you stop dieting and proceed with your life as you once did, you will gain back the weight. Despite its obviosity, most people are oblivious to the fact that maintaining weight loss is harder than losing it in the first place. To lose the weight and keep it off, one has to change the habits that caused gaining it in the first place. Albert Einstein said, "Insanity is doing the same thing over and over again and expecting different results." That also applies to maintaining weight loss.

Thus, to maintain weight loss people have to change their old lifestyle and adopt a new one, with new habits and patterns, not just physical but also mental, spiritual and emotional. Mental health is an important factor that plays a major role in organizing our lives and maintaining our physical and emotional wellbeing. It helps us accept ourselves and prevents us from comparing ourselves with others. It is also what keeps our sanity despite social media. It is what protects us from getting caught in the loop that drives us back to our old bad habits. Once we are back to the old habits, we will gain the weight we lost and maybe more.

Unfortunately, fat cells are always active. They shrink, but they never disappear. Once you lose weight, fat cells shrink. When you start eating again, they enlarge and become more active, just like a person who had been starved for days would behave when you take him to an open buffet. Once you start feeding them, and in fear of being starved again, fat cells will multiply quickly to store more body fat, resulting in more weight gain. This is one of the reasons why the yo-yo diet is a disaster. Yo-yo dieting is the process of dieting to lose weight, gaining it back, then dieting agan to lose it, and repeating the process over and over again. It has long term harmful results on the body.

For this reason, changing your style and eating habits is all you need to live a normal life, achieve results without killing yourself in the gym, starving and depriving yourself from eating the food you like. Small changes over time add up, and by accomplishing them, you will live a much better life, a happier one with less stress and anxiety. It is better to lose 10 kg over a period of one year than in a month. This gives you plenty of time during which you can eat properly without having to starve. You will be surprised at how much more you can enjoy life consuming 1900/2000 calories per day instead of 1000/1200. Obviously, the progress of weight loss slows down, but this gives you the chance to eat a variety of food, add more carbs, more protein, more fat.

When I adjusted my calorie intake to 2300/2500 per day, that gave me the opportunity to enjoy life better, go out with my friend for dinners, and at the same time lose weight slowly, and enjoy the process rather than being frustrated about it. I did not deprive myself from food, just reduced my portions. I paid attention to what I ate and watched how I consumed my calories. If I surpassed 2500 calories in a day, the following day I dropped the calories to 2000 or 2100, but that was it. That is the whole concept.

I do not want to be eating salads until eternity. I do not want to fast for 10 hours and then eat only salads and proteins for two hours, without carbs. Two weeks of this routine can wear you out, guaranteed. You will eventually lose it, you will mess up a day and before you know it, you have gained more weight than when you started the diet.

You lose the momentum not because you are a loser or a failure, but because this is not a normal life to live. It is as simple as that. If you can manage to live it for a month or two (I lived it for four years), you will not be able to live it for 30 or 40 years. And even if you could sustain it for this long, you will not be living a normal life. I am not talking here about people who this lifestyle is their normal, I am talking about people who are struggling with their weight. With continuous dieting, you will lose your hair because your body is not receiving the right amounts of nutrients it needs. It will also increase your anxiety and stress and leave you miserable at times. Moreover, continuous dieting will drop your productivity, due to the exhaustion from excessive exercise and nutrients deficiency. This will negatively affect and impact your work, health, social life and relations.

Losing weight and maintaining it is first and foremost a lifestyle that one has to work hard to acquire and maintain. Remember, it is your body, your journey, your life. Others have different lives and jobs than you. They do not have your variables either. It is unrealistic and unfair to compare yourself to anyone else. You have to accept yourself for who you are. It is also important to understand and believe that being overweight or obese does not make you a bad person, or that your life sucks. It only indicates that you need small changes and adjustments in your life, that in time, and with patience and perseverance will show great results.

The most valuable lesson I have learned throughout my transformational journey to date is that small changes over a longer period of time achieve better and sustainable results than trying to accomplish big changes over a short period of time. Big changes and quick results did not last. It became inevitable that I had to have midcourse corrections, and approach my next phase with a new strategy. Losing weight is no longer my long-term plan, but rather sustaining the weight loss and living a healthy life. Without the stress and anxiety of dieting, I am more focused, more productive. I eat better. I eat whatever I want. I go out with my friends. And I lost most of the weight I gained and I am maintaining it. I don't have six packs yet, but believe me when I say I am much happier. In brief, I feel good.

That is what should be done. No one journey fits all. The longer we travel, the journey unfolds and evolves.

IT'S NOT THE END OF THE JOURNEY, BUT THE BEGINNING OF A NEW ONE.

At some point in my life I thought there was no need for me in this world. I really wanted to die, to disappear from the face of earth. Perhaps fall in a black hole and vanish. I hated every single moment of my pathetic life. I didn't want to get out of bed in the morning. I didn't want to go to school or go to training. I didn't want to do anything, except hide in my room. I felt I was useless and that I will pity myself until I die, disappear or be abducted by aliens and get lost in a faraway galaxy. I made no difference in anyone's life. My presence or absence didn't impact anyone enough to care. No one enjoyed my company or noticed my absence. For many years, I felt alone and unwanted.

After losing the weight, gaining it back and trying to lose it one more time, I realized I was not alone. Along the process, I became aware that it wasn't just about me. Many people around me were influenced, impacted and affected by my transformation journey. I have influenced and changed the lives of many; my trainees, people I talked to in person or those who watched my YouTube video. The realization of having a bigger purpose in life cured me from depression. It cured me from many emotional and mental ailments. I tell people when you have a bigger purpose, your problems look smaller. That's why I wrote this book.

I wrote this book for people who feel different because society had put them in a certain box, especially the overweight and obese one, because I feel their struggles. Even if they try to conceal their pain and pretend they are not bothered by the challenges and struggles they are going through, or that obesity is not affecting their lives, I know deep down they are unhappy. I see and feel their pain. I have been there and I know exactly how it feels. It takes one to understand another. I went through the same pain and I understand the anger, frustration and despair of every obese person out there. I want people who see themselves not fit or not good enough by society standards, to change their mindset.

If you are suffering from social labeling and going through emotional and mental struggles because of that, don't let people's behaviors and attitudes decide for you how to live your life. It is not easy to brush their unkindness, harsh words and vile stares off your shoulder, but it is important to understand that you are the only one who can set the rules of your life. See and accept yourself in the image you want to see. Like yourself as you are. Don't let anyone put you in their boxes or make you feel inferior because you don't fit their mould. Don't allow anyone to make you feel you are insignificant.

I just have one thing to say after all I went through and witnessed; every diet works, every exercise works, every step you take towards losing weight works. Walking will help you burn calories, jogging will help you lose weight, green tea will burn the fat, even eating McDonalds will make you lose weight. There is no such a thing as good food or bad food for dieting. There is a calorie deficit and that's why diets work. If you want to lose weight fast and you feel this is what you want to do, do it. Just learn how to maintain it and know that it's not an endless process. If you have the ability and the patience to lose weight gradually, do it.

Every path is different; every human is different. Because it worked for others, it doesn't mean it will work for you. Conversely, because it didn't work for others, it doesn't mean it will not work for you. Many other factors are involved, and we don't share the same ones. Just do it. Don't think about the challenges and failures you are going to encounter on your path. You will fail 100 times. Get up and try again.

This should not come as a surprise to you, but your diet is not going to work from the first time. You can try twice, three times, ten times and perhaps start losing weight after ten failed trials or even more. Even after eating a large burger with fries and soda, get back up and try again. It is okay. You are only human. If you are persistent enough, one day you will make it. It is as simple as that.

There is no magic formula or secret ingredient to losing weight.

You want a support system to help and motivate you, good for you. You want to do tricks to help you eat less, like using smaller plates to decrease your calories intake, or throwing out junk food to avoid temptations, good for you. But at the end, the desire to lose weight comes from within. If you have this desire you will eventually lose it no matter what people say.

If you seek a purpose and you want to help people to lose weight, you will stop looking at yourself as useless, and you will start working towards the goal of helping others. When you choose this path, you will find yourself losing weight and getting in shape to become a role model for others. This is just an example, but at the end what it boils down to is, you have the power and the will in your hands. Even if you decide one day you want to undergo surgery to lose weight, cut half of your stomach or follow whatever trend is going on, it doesn't mean you are a failure, or you don't know how to do it. You just took a different path.

I chose the title of the book "I am not Fat" for the following reason. We are not caricatures. We are humans. We have emotions, weaknesses and insecurities, but also have dreams and want our lives to mean something. We want to love and be loved. We want to be accepted by society for who we are. The whole package; not just our exterior shell. But first, we must accept ourselves for who we are. The good and the not so good.
The whole package. At the end of the journey there is inner peace. This will not be achieved, however, without self acceptance. Live the life you want to live and don't let anyone dictate to you how to live it. You are perfect just the way you are, don't let anyone convince you otherwise. I truly believe in me and believe in you and I wish you all the success in the world. At the end of your journey I hope you reach your inner peace.

This is the message I wanted to convey, my only purpose to write this book. I hope you found value in it and if affected your life in a positive way.

APPENDIX

WHAT SWAT TAUGHT ME

Through SWAT, I gained valuable real life business lessons and first hand experiences. And because experiences come with a price, I also learned from SWAT's mistakes and how to avoid them. Here are some of the problems that hindered the growth of the business and eventually led to its collapse. They could be applied to any business.

1- Business Model: We didn't have a clear business model or understood the one we created correctly. We earned money, but didn't know how to spend it effectively to grow and develop the business. We didn't stop to think if it was better for us or not to have our own place and pay rent instead of going to gyms and negotiate a deal with them. We were content to just take a percentage or a commission. The operation was risk free, but we weren't actually growing, in a sense that if we made 10,000 LE, the gym collected half of that. If we made 100,000, the gym's cut was 50,000. While there was no risk, our expenses grew in parallel with the growth of the business.

2- Customer Service: We didn't understand what it meant to have recurrent customers, or how to keep customers coming back. Customers were the most important stakeholders of our business. Without them, we had no business, yet, we didn't understand the importance of customer satisfaction, or why we had to keep pampering them to keep coming back.

All we cared about was to fill the 15 spots we had in the class. Old customers, new customers, it didn't matter, as long as these 15 spots were filled. Recurrent customers like to feel special, but we treated them just like the one-timers. We gave them no incentives to renew their membership. What saved us at the beginning was that we offered innovative, enjoyable and effective workouts. They came back because they enjoyed the training and liked our spirit, because we loved what we did and our positive energy reflected on them. But we didn't keep track of them. We didn't have their contact info. If customers left or fell sick, we really didn't care about them. Customer experience was not our forte, mind you were still 17-years-olds, who never worked before. But our spirits and energy were high and that helped us grow slowly.

3- Process Documentation: We didn't document anything. We didn't know our numbers. How much did we make? No one knew. How much money did we make from this branch this month? No one knew. How many clients did we have this month? No one knew. The business operation was chaotic and messy. We opened the drawer, found the money we made and divided it, and we were good. We didn't keep track of anything. We had no records to indicate if we were actually growing or declining.

4- Marketing: We had no marketing plan. Marketing became an issue of conflict between us. Zeyad and I believed marketing is a 24/7 process, and that we should have continuous marketing campaigns going on at all times, even if some lacked the wow factor. We had to continuously motivate people and share testimonials from the clients.

Karim on the other hand didn't want to exert any time, money or effort in marketing. He believed releasing one video per year like the transformational one was enough. With Yehia under Karim's spell, we were stuck with their mentalities and couldn't do much about it.

No matter how much we tried, Karim insisted he was right and everyone else wrong. He refused to listen to any of my suggestions. We were neither able to document the business nor market it properly. I realized I spent more time arguing with my partners than actually solving any of the business problems. We weren't moving forward because the partners weren't compatible. Even though we were good friends, we had different business orientations. We were not on the same wavelength. Karim was a very toxic person and on the other hand, I was too passive. I didn't hold my position. As long as things were moving, I didn't want to rock the boat. I ignored the problems when they surfaced, which I shouldn't have done. I should have fought harder to get my point across.

*

ENTREPRENEURIAL LESSONS

1- Understand your business model and how you are going to make money. What are the sources of your revenue and how are you going to spend it?

2- Document everything, every little thing, and understand your numbers. If someone asks for the cost of customer acquisition, you should know the number. If someone asks for the expected lifetime value of your customers, you should know the answer.

3- Understand your marketing strategy. How are you getting into the market? What's the purpose of your marketing campaigns? Understand your campaigns from A to Z and always have a marketing campaign going on. You market to acquire new customers. You market to keep your existing customers coming back. You market to persuade those who are sitting on the fence to take action and buy something from you. It is important to understand these business aspects. Business is not just money coming in. Every pound comes from a different way. You have to understand how this pound came in and how to grow it to become 10 pounds. In our era, learning digital marketing is as important as breathing, sleeping and eating.

4- Customers make or break your business. They are the most important factor in your business and thus it is equally important to understand and create a customer experience for it. Customers come to you, either to solve their problem or because they want to be pampered. You have to solve their problems and pamper them. If you can do that, you guarantee their loyalty. No one could expand their business without taking good care of their customers.

5- My last advice is to choose your partners wisely. Because they are your best childhood friends and you know everything about each other, doesn't mean they can be good business partners. A business partner is someone who can support you. Your partners' strength should be your weakness and vice-versa so you become a team, a strong force, that between both of you, you drive a strong business.

Looking back at SWAT, I believe these were the mistakes that led it to its shutdown.

ACKNOWLEDGMENTS

Writing a book is harder than I thought and more rewarding than I could have ever imagined. None of this would have been possible without the support and encouragement of Nour, my best friend and coworker. He was the first person I trained in my life. We became best friends ever since. He was also the first to know I was writing a book. He supported and encouraged me endlessly. Thank you Nour for taking some work off my shoulders to give me more time to work on the book.

I am really grateful for Karim, Zeyad and Yehia for building SWAT with me. It was a hell of a journey and I cherish every moment of it, the good and the bad. Thank you Yehia for also helping me bring this book to life.

Special thanks to Alexandra Kinias, my editor. I cannot appreciate enough her constant support and amazing input. Thank you for your encouragement, efforts and hard work and most importantly for helping me finish the book. I am really grateful for such an amazing journey.

Although this period of my life was filled with many ups and downs, Sharabasy and Fady were always there for me. They knew how to cheer me up and bring a smile to my face. For that I am very thankful. Also huge thanks to Aly Ramzy and Yomna for creating such an amazing book cover.

To all my friends and everyone who I met and impacted my life in any way, thank you. I really appreciate everything you have done for me. This book wouldn't have been complete without you.,

ABE SOLYMAN

---

[1] Street Workout the Art of Transformation

www.ingramcontent.com/pod-product-compliance
Lightning Source LLC
Chambersburg PA
CBHW032042090426
42744CB00004B/89